The X Rays

Frederick Strange Kolle

REPRESSED
PUBLISHING

ISBN: 978-1-5222-0328-5

Printed in the United States of America
Repressed Publishing LLC
Provo, Utah

ISBN 978-1-5222-0328-5

www.RepressedPublishing.com

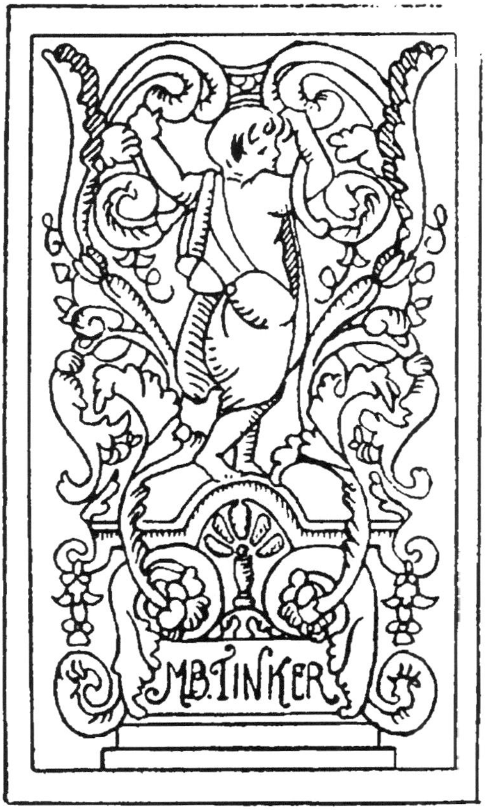
M.B. TINKER

THE X RAYS.

THEIR PRODUCTION AND APPLICATION.

BY

FREDERICK STRANGE KOLLE, M. D.,

Radiographer to the Methodist Episcopal Hospital; Member of the Kings' County Medical Society, the Brooklyn Pathological Society, the Long Island College Hospital, and Kings' County Hospital Alumni Association, of Brooklyn, N. Y.

NEW YORK:
J. S. OGILVIE PUBLISHING COMPANY,
57 ROSE STREET.

"LIGHT—MORE LIGHT."

TO

PROFESSOR WILHELM KONRAD ROENTGEN,

THE DISCOVERER OF

A NEW FORM OF RADIATION,

BY WHICH THE ENTIRE SCIENTIFIC WORLD HAS PROFITED,

THIS VOLUME IS HUMBLY DEDICATED

BY THE AUTHOR.

PREFACE.

In the present volume it has been the specific aim of the author to present to the reader, student and surgeon a concise and demonstrative treatise on the use and value of Professor Roentgen's discovery. Although the discovery has hardly ceased to be a novelty, it has nevertheless taken a deserving place among the approved and accepted aids to diagnosis and record.

As all knowledge is derived from original research, it has been found advisable to bring the reader in touch and harmony with some of those valuable results and inferences that have been recorded from time to time by the experiments of noted scientists, especially those that have remained with us, acting as landmarks, as it were, in the progress of this science.

In lieu of the fact that this subject dates back to the original research of electrical discharge, it has been deemed necessary to acquaint the reader with those results which led directly to the discovery of the X rays.

The subject matter is divided into Part I., which contains a compact description of Electricity, its uses and application in connection with the subject; and Part II., treating of the practical and theoretical advance and application of Radiography.

As the field of experiments and record is necessarily extensive, inasmuch as the discovery aroused world-wide interest, the author has deducted the results recorded, here and abroad, in standard and accepted works, and of reliable and authoritative scientists, to whom great credit is due—while in giving his own knowledge of the subject, he endeavors to aid the amateur and specialist in the advancement of this new and valuable branch of science.

Results and cross-references to other works and experimenters are credited by number, referred to in footnotes, wherein it has been the author's earnest desire to exclude all criticism of any particular work or result, or to deal personally with any one experimenter.

The volume is a simple record of the pioneer work of the advancements in this science. The compiler has endeavored to combine all that bears importance, originality, and is worthy of preservation, and begs to offer his thanks to the many medical men who have favored him with the opportunity of making, and permitting the reproduction of, radiograms of cases under their special charge.

F. S. K.

BROOKLYN, N. Y., Dec., 1897.

CONTENTS.

PART I.

PART II.

PART I.

Electricity—Its Uses and Application in Connection with Radiography.

THE X RAYS.

PART I.

CHAPTER I.

THE nature of electricity in itself is a property of which little is practically known; it is, however, conceded by many that the characteristics of polarity, or the to and fro property it has, is due to molecular motion. The manifestation of such is chiefly attraction and repulsion, but is also recognized by its power of decomposing chemical compounds; by its power to produce heat and light; and lastly may be evidenced by its violent action.

Electricity may be divided into several divisions.

I. Magnetism. II. Frictional electricity. III. Dynamical electricity. IV. Animal electricity. V. Thermal electricity.

I.

Magnets may be classified as A, Natural; B, Artificial; and C, Electro-magnets.

A.

Magnetism is observed naturally in a certain form of iron ore named loadstone, first discovered by the Greeks in the town of Magnesia, Lydia, and later in Norway and

Sweden. Chemically it is known as a magnetic oxide of iron.

B.

Artificial magnets were discovered by Coloumb in 1802. They were made of hardened steel to which the magnetism was imparted by rubbing its surface with that of the natural magnet, constantly following the one direction. These are called *permanent*. *Temporary* magnets are made of soft iron, but do not retain their magnetism when the exciting cause is removed.

The magnet we are most accustomed to seeing is that in the form of a horseshoe or the needle of the compass. It is well known that the magnet has two poles, north and south (N. and S.), and that a bar of magnetized iron will attract metal objects at either end; but if the north or positive is brought in contact with the same end of another magnet, the attraction at once ceases and we have repulsion.

This proves that we have two unlike poles—one that attracts while the other repels. These poles are described as positive and negative, north and south. (Fig. 1.)

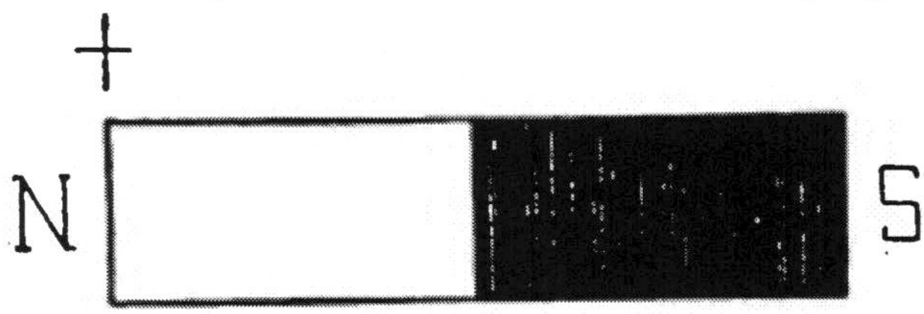

FIG. 1.

Now we may transmit this magnetism by induction by presenting a small piece of iron, in the form of a nail or ring, to one pole of the magnet. It will be found by applying another ring to the one already attracted, that it will remain suspended from the first one, showing that the iron ring has become magnetized by induction. (See Fig. 2.)

This induction goes on to a third, fourth, and so on, as long as the first ring remains suspended. Where considerable power is required of a magnet, it has been found necessary to place several magnets side by side; these will

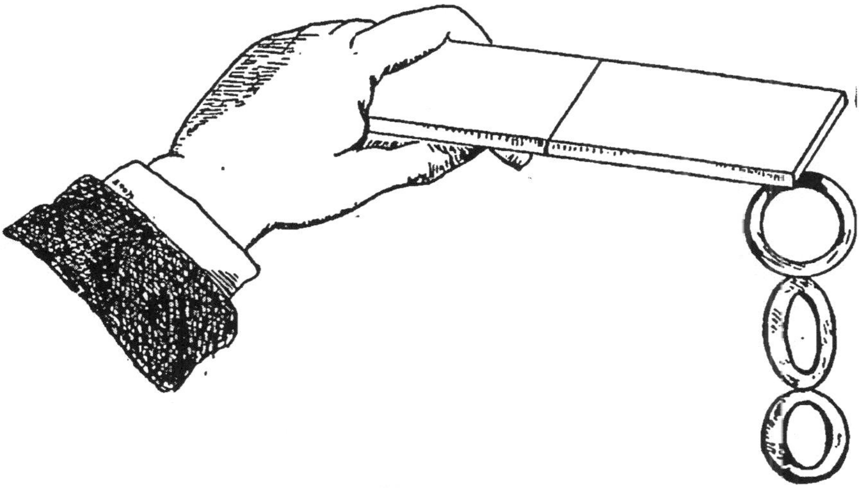

FIG. 2.

attract a piece of iron, called in this case the Armature, very forcibly to its free ends or poles. This collection of magnets is called a Magnetic Battery. (Fig. 3.)

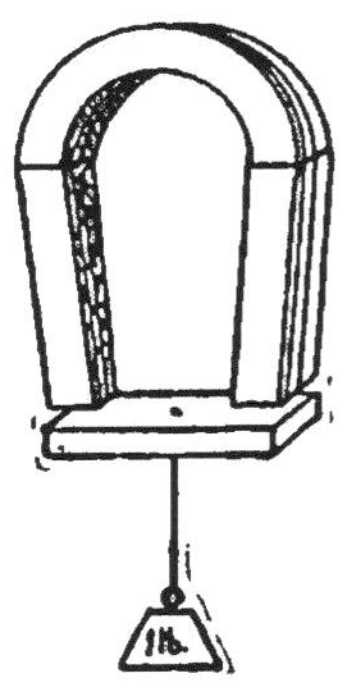

FIG. 3.

Bodies not attracted by magnetism are said to be diamagnetic, such as gold, silver, bismuth, lead, copper, etc.

C.

There is another form of magnet, and that is the Electro-magnet.

If a bar of soft iron, bent in the form of a horseshoe, is wound at either end with a silk-covered insulated wire, and a current of electricity allowed to pass through these coils, it will be found that the iron has become magnetized and will attract the armature very forcibly. If the current is broken the armature falls, showing that the magnetism is gone. (Fig. 4.)

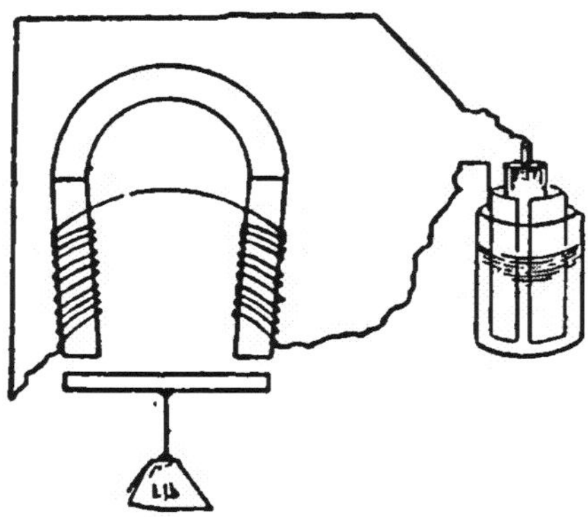

FIG. 4.

If a bar of soft iron is wound over with silk-covered wire in the form of a Solenoid, and a current of an electric battery is allowed to pass through the wire, the same thing is observed. The current makes a magnet of the conductor by bringing about or inducing a whirl of lines of magnetic force around it, as well as in its own helix. Orsted, in 1819,[1] in this way discovered the Galvanoscope. This was made by placing a magnetic needle set upon a pivot between the two ends of a piece of iron, and charging the iron with an electric current; the needle at once deflects or deviates in the opposite direction to that of the current.

1 Wildermann's "Grundlehre der Elektricität," p. 65.

If now the intensity of the current is increased, the needle will deflect still more. (Fig. 5.)

Ampere completed the greater portion of the discovery of the electro-magnet. The following is the law (Ampere's),[2] as given by him, to determine the direction of these lines of induced magnetic force. He supposed an observer lying down upon the wire, along which a current flows, the current entering at his feet and going out at the head. Then if he faced the needle he would at once see that the

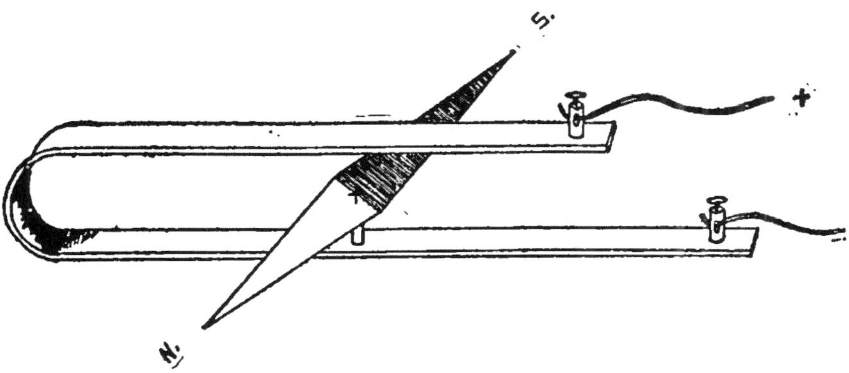

Fig. 5.

north pole of the needle had deviated toward his left hand. Whereupon Ampere established the following principles:

1. Magnets exercise a directive force upon currents.

2. The earth, which acts like a great magnet upon a magnetic needle, acts in the same manner upon movable currents; in other words, it directs the current so that it is perpendicular to the plane coinciding with the magnetic meridian.

3. The free wires of two like currents attract each other when their currents *flow* in the same direction, and repel each other when their currents *flow* in opposite directions.

2 "Ganot's Physics," Peck, p. 480.

4. An Ampere solenoid, suspended by its steel points in cups of mercury placed one above the other, arranged as in Fig. 6, through which a current is passed, will

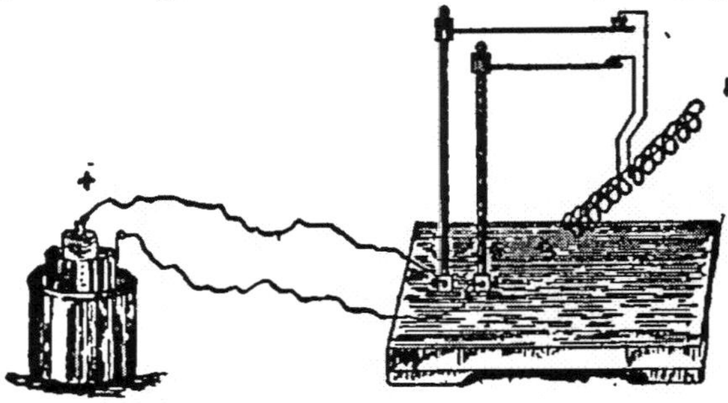

FIG. 6.

arrange itself in the meridian exactly like that of a magnetic needle.

Ampere believes magnetism to be due to currents of electricity flowing around the ultimate molecules of a magnet, arranging themselves in a meridian exactly like that of a magnetic needle. His theory of magnetism is as follows: He supposes magnetism to be due to currents of electricity forming around ultimate molecules of a magnet, always in the same direction. The currents in

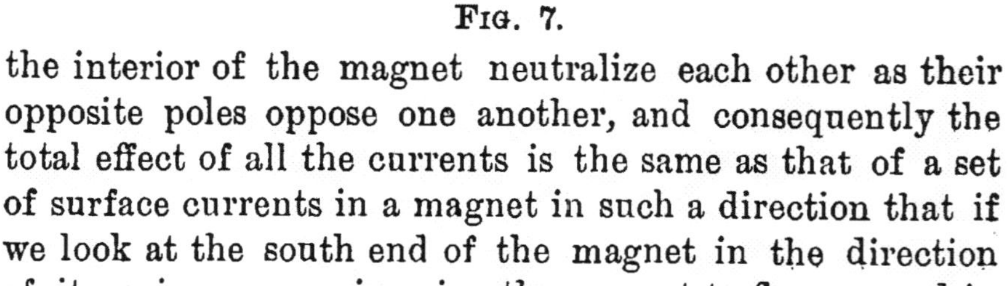

FIG. 7.

the interior of the magnet neutralize each other as their opposite poles oppose one another, and consequently the total effect of all the currents is the same as that of a set of surface currents in a magnet in such a direction that if we look at the south end of the magnet in the direction of its axis, we may imagine the current to flow around in the same direction as the hands of a clock. (See Fig.

Not only is the magnetism observed in the conductor placed within the coil of wire, but also in the solenoid surrounding it; but only in a very moderate degree as compared to that of the two combined, when soft iron is used as a conductor.

Soft iron is claimed to increase the magnetic effect under proper conditions as much as 32.8 times. The combined

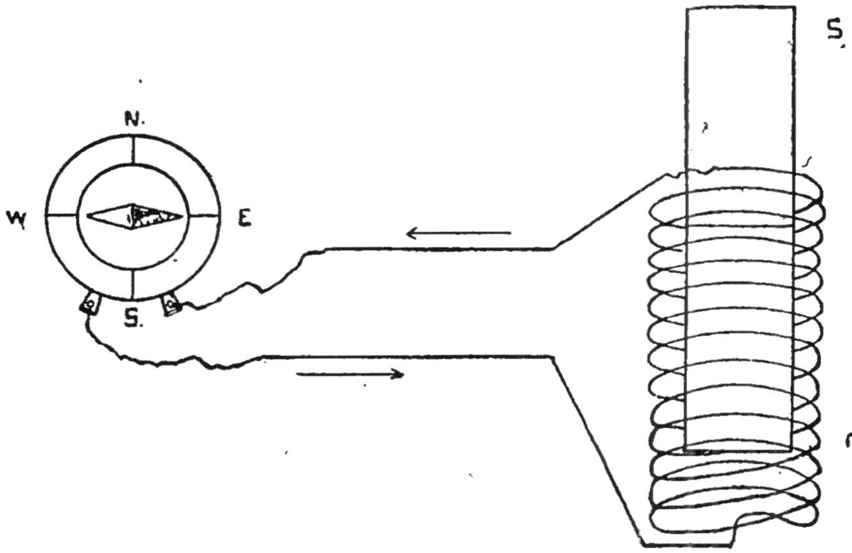

FIG. 8.

form of such magnet, *i.e.*, a conductor and solenoid, is called an electro-magnet.

If we connect the terminals of a coil of insulated wire wound upon a bobbin to the Galvanometer as described, or to one not so simple in construction as Nobilis's Multiplicater, and introduce a bar magnet into the helix of the former, a momentary current is induced, as shown by the deflection of the needle in an opposite direction. (Fig. 8.

If a permanent magnet is placed so that the coil can be raised and lowered at will, the same phenomenon will be noticed—namely, a to and fro induced current. The solenoid in the above figure acts the same as the conductor or magnet, showing that the properties of each are subject to the same law of attraction and repulsion.

II.

FRICTIONAL ELECTRICITY.

About five hundred years B.C. Thales of Miletus[3] observed the attractional phenomenon exhibited by amber when briskly rubbed with wool. Light pieces of paper, straws and such like were easily attracted. At the end of the sixteenth century William Gilbert, an English physician, discovered that a number of other substances, such as resin, silver, silks, etc., acquired the same attractive power, when being rubbed with cat skin.

This experiment can be easily demonstrated by briskly rubbing a hard rubber penholder over a coat sleeve for a moment, and bringing it in the neighborhood of little pieces of fuzzy blotting paper, when they will be made to jump from the table to the holder, and cling to it for several seconds at a time.

This is called frictional or static electricity. A very simple experiment for showing this phenomenon is the electroscope, which consists of a glass rod mounted on a wooden base and capped at its upper extremity with a metal ball, which holds a fine wire. From the end of this wire, a small ball of elder pith is suspended by the aid of a fine silken thread.

To find out if the body rubbed was electrified, it was only necessary to present it near the pith ball, which, if electrified, would be attracted to it, otherwise nothing would occur. If now we rub a piece of resin briskly with flannel and present it to the pith ball, it will fly away from it, or toward another body presented, which we will say was a glass rod, previously rubbed with silk. This shows that there are two kinds of electricity—the same as in the magnet having two poles, like and unlike, so it is here. We have resinous electricity as a result of rubbing the

---

3 Peck, "Ganot's Physics," p. 420.

resin with flannel, which may here be termed negative (—), and the other vitreous electricity obtained by rubbing glass with silk, called positive (+); the former repels and the latter attracts.

Here the electricity, whether positive or negative, depends upon the substance rubbed, and the nature of the substance with which it is rubbed. The relative position of these substances is given by Ganot as follows:

Positive (+): Catskin, glass, ivory, silk, rock crystal, wood, flannel, shellac, rubber, gutta percha, metals. Negative (—): When any of these electrified bodies are brought in contact with a body oppositely charged, the forces in the two are at once discharged and become neutral toward each other. If, however, there remains a space between the two, and if the charge in each is high, the accumulated potential will allow the discharge to jump across the space from positive to negative, and as both are discharged at once there will be a spark or an electrical flash observed between the ends of the electrified bodies.

Several machines for producing this form of electricity have been made. The simplest was that of Volta, called the Electrophor; but the earliest hand friction machine was invented about two hundred years ago by Otto von Guericke and consisted of a ball of sulphur fixed upon a wooden axis. Upon turning the axis and holding one hand against the sulphur ball, a quantity of electricity was developed. One made by Winter,[4] both simple and which produced considerable discharge, was constructed as follows: It consisted of a large glass plate mounted upon an insulated shaft at its axis; a conductor with two or three rings of dry wood at its extremity, and a frictional arrangement at the opposite side, with its conductor. A system of conductors was added to the conductor containing the rings, in the

4 "Elektrisier Maschine von Winter," Grundlehre der Elektricität, part I., chap. II. Wildermann.

form of three hollow brass spheres, mounted upon a glass base.

At the extremity of the opposite conductor, one large brass sphere was mounted upon a glass rod. The wooden rings had on their inner surface a groove, in which a number of fine pegs of brass were inserted on a level with the ring surface; these were placed directly opposite to each other on either side of the glass plate.

The frictional arrangement of the other, or opposite side, consisted of a leather-polstered fork of wood, that came in close opposition with the glass plate on either side. These leather polsters or cushions were amalgamated with a mixture composed as follows: tin, one part; zinc, one part; and mercury, two parts. A protecting shield made of waxed-paper was placed over the lower part of the whole to protect the plate from air as much as possible. The negative conductor was connected with the earth by means of a chain.

If the handle of the shaft of this machine be turned in a direction resembling the movements of clock hands, a friction would be caused between the glass and amalgam of the leather cushions. The glass will be electrified positively, while the cushion receives a negative charge.

The positive electricity of the plate would be received or discharged by meeting with the brass pegs of the wooden rings, and so neutralized for another charge, whereas the negative was discharged by way of the chain to the earth; this is continued as the plate is rapidly turned—the positive electricity is stored by the balls which act as accumulators, storing the positive electricity collected as described, so becoming the positive conductor. In this way considable positive and negative current may be accumulated at will. The word accumulator is used in the sense of a condenser.

By a condenser is meant an apparatus employed for

the accumulation of electricity. They are of various forms, but may briefly be described as two conductors separated by an insulated material.

One of the simplest is that in the form of a leyden jar. The jar is made by taking a wide-mouthed thin glass jar, not quite covered inside and outside with tin foil, fastened by the use of shellac varnish. A cover of hardwood is placed within the mouth, through the center of which is passed a wire connected to the tin foil within the jar

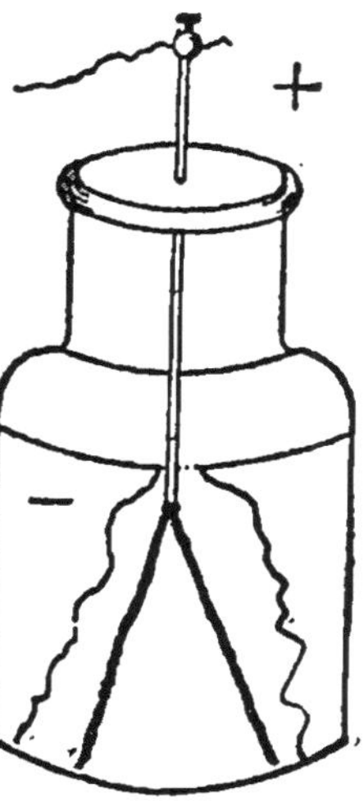

Fig. 9.

and having a small brass ball at its other extremity. It is charged by holding the outer tinned part in the hand, and the ball or button in contact with the positive conductor of an electrical machine. The positive (+) electricity is accumulated in the inner tinned surface and acts by induction upon the outer coating, which becomes negative as the positive is carried away by the hand, through the body. To discharge such a condenser, all that is necessary is to hold the jar with one hand over the tinned outer surface, and bring the other in contact with the metal ball or button, when the sensation of shock is at once perceived in the arms and body, immediately devoiding the jar of its current and returning it to its natural state.

If a wire insulated for the hand at the middle be applied in like manner, a spark will be drawn from the ball, and no shock perceived. If a number of these leyden jars are connected, they act like a single conductor.

Professor Holtz, of Berlin, invented another form of machine which he called the influence machine, based upon the principle of continuous induction. This has two glass plates, one being fixed and the other made to revolve; the electricity is collected by metallic combs, etc.

The machine will be referred to later. It gives a torrent of sparks, but is readily affected by the moisture in the air; but as compared with the former it is much better, the length of the spark produced being almost that of the radius of the revolving plate.

CHAPTER II.

VOLTAIC OR CHEMICAL ELECTRICITY.

THIS is the most important of the divisions of electricity and will be thoroughly described.

Chemical electricity may be said to be of two kinds—primary and secondary; its source being that of a battery, so called.

Volta showed that if two heterogeneous metals were brought in contact, electricity was exhibited. When two pieces of unlike metal, or one metal and the other a non-metallic substance, were placed in a solution called electrolyte, both pieces having conductors attached to them, and the latter were connected outside of the liquid, a current was noted.

This idea was advanced by Professor Galvani, and the above immersion of two pieces of unlike metal into an electrolyte was called the Galvanic Cell, in honor of the discoverer. The relation of the metals to each other when brought in contact was about as follows: Positive (+), zinc, lead, tin, iron, copper, silver, gold, platinum and carbon. Negative (—).

After considerable experimenting, Volta originated the so-called Volta's column or pile. (Fig. 10.)

This was composed of an upright stand made of three glass columns 40 centimeters high, ending in a wooden base and top; a number of metal plates composed of zinc and copper, one of each soldered together, and lastly a number of cloth plaques, rendered slightly moist by some acid solution. The metal plates were placed between the upright columns as per illustration—zinc at the bottom and copper at the top; then a layer of cloth and so on upward, until the entire number had been placed. It was thus observed that, by this contact method, a chemical reaction would take place, and by the use of the electroscope

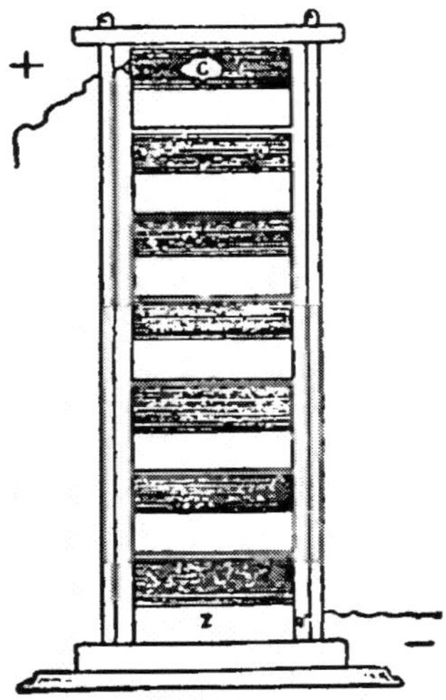

FIG. 10.

the negative was found to be the zinc, and the positive the copper end.

However, the contact theory was soon banished by the discovery of the chemical cell, the simplest form of which was made as follows:

A plate of copper and zinc were partially immersed in a solution of sulphuric acid and water, and each plate was connected to a wire which led out of the cell. If these wires were connected, a decomposition of the solution took place, forming hydrogen at the copper plate, and oxygen at the zinc plate, combining with the zinc plate to form zinc sulphate.

This is known as electrolysis or decomposition of water. It was also found that the zinc was negative (—) and the copper positive (+), moving in the course of the arrow in the illustration. (Fig. 11.)

The chemical reaction in the cell was said to be due to a division and re-formation of the molecules of the conductors, *i.e.*, the positive would remove a molecule from the solution, at the same time giving one of its own to the outleading wire; the liquid in turn would take a molecule away from the negative metal, which in turn would receive one from the leading-in wire, and so on.

This leads us to understand that electricity is developed

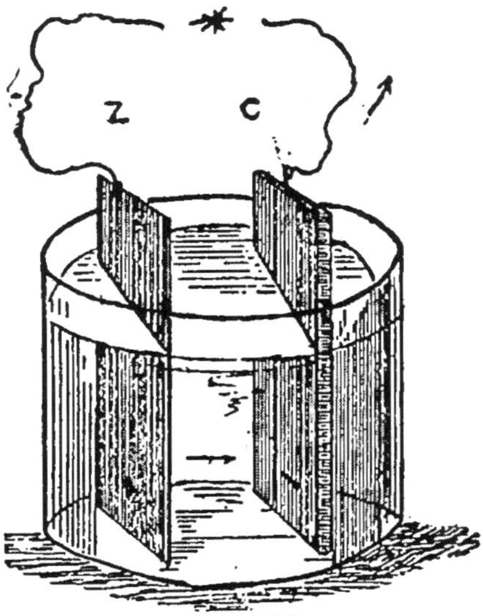

FIG. 11.

by chemical action and flows from the zinc plate, passes through the liquid to the copper plate, and outward to the external conductor; therefore we say that electricity flows from the positive pole outside the liquid or cell, and returns by the negative plate within the liquid, from which the electricity flows; for this reason it is called the positive element, and the other plate which carries it out is called the negative element. (Fig. 11.)

The illustration constitutes the voltaic primary cell, of

which we have a great number of varieties; some of the most useful will be described in Chapter III.

The current flow or circuit is said to be closed when the wires are connected, and there is a constant flow of the electricity through the wires.

The circuit is open when the wires are disconnected, hindering the outflow of force.

Poles or electrodes are the wires connected to the plates of the cell, the positive (+) pole is connected to the negative plate, and the negative pole to the positive plate.

To ground a battery is to connect the external conductor of the battery to the earth, so causing a neutral state of the cell elements.

A battery may be termed a cell, or a collection of two or more cells. By elements we mean the separate parts or plates of the cell, *i.e.*, the zinc element, the carbon element, etc.

The most difficult things to grasp and understand in electricity are the terms, their meaning and uses. It has always been a bugbear with the beginner, and the bewildering ways in which electro-motive force (E. M. F.), potential, volt, ampere, ohm, coloumb, capacity, farad, micro-farad and watts are thrust at the student is not only bewildering, but unkind.

ELECTRICAL POTENTIAL.

I will endeavor to make these points clear to the reader. *Electrical Potential*, tension, or electro-motive force expressed thus (E. M. F.), is that property of a body by means of which electricity tends to pass from it and flow to another body. For example, if a body of water were placed at an elevated area—say a hill, and if a chute were made leading it downhill to the ocean, the water would acquire a certain amount of power to do work, in its course downward, or in other words has acquired potential force in rushing downhill, turning water wheels, machinery, etc.

Electricity is a force, not a substance, and is constantly trying to reach an equilibrium. If now there is considerable electricity in the cell, the same as the water on the hill, the current has a tendency to rush out to overcome the places less charged, and in so doing acquires force, tension, or potential. The greater the quantity at one end, the greater the tension to overcome the difference at the other end.

Electricity, although not a substance and not having length nor breadth, can be measured, and the unit of electrical pressure is called the volt.

The *Volt* is that power which the electric current possesses to overcome resistance. It is a pressure about equal to that given by the Daniell cell.

As you know, water pressure can be measured, so can electricity. Electrical pressure is measured not as water is in pounds, but by volts.

RESISTANCE AND CONDUCTORS.

It has been shown that the water running downhill has acquired a certain amount of potential to do work; so has it acquired a force to overcome the resistance offered by the water wheel to drive the wheels of a mill.

The force necessary to drive the wheel and its dependent machinery, is the resistance which the water has to overcome, and the heavier the work of the machinery the greater will the resistance be, and so is it with electricity.

Electricity, as you know, is propagated by conductors made of metal, preferably of copper, as that is cheap and a better conductor than iron or some other metal, and for another reason—the better the conductor the less the resistance.

The conductors in electricity are usually made in the form of copper wire.

The resistance of electricity is the opposition which the current has to overcome. The resistance of a conductor depends upon three things: first, its power of conduction or conductivity; second, its cross section; and third, its length. The less the conducting power the greater the resistance; the greater the cross section the less the resistance; the greater the length the greater the resistance; or in other words, a large and short wire offers less obstruction than a long and thin wire.

In electricity there are two forms of resistance: internal, or that within the cell offered by the liquid conductor between the two plates, and the external, or that resistance offered by the conductor outside the cell.

But the internal resistance, which is considerably greater than that of metal, does not interest us so much as the external; however, the internal and external resistances should be equal to get the best results.

THE OHM.

The unit of resistance is called the *Ohm.* It is the resistance offered to the passage of the current by a column of mercury one square millimeter in cross section and 106 centimeters in length.

The ohm permits a current to flow through a conductor at the rate of one ampere, under the pressure of one volt. It will be advisable to refer to the following law, called Ohm's Law: "The strength of a current developed by a battery will be equal to the electro-motive force (E. M. F.) divided by the resistance. This is stated algebraically thus:

$$C = \frac{E.M.F.}{R' + R}$$

It is evident that in order to increase the value of C or current, in the formula, we must increase the E. M. F. or diminish the R (resistance). If we wish to increase the electro-motive force (E. M.F.) we must select such metals and solutions as will give high intensity, or we may join several cells, so that the force of one is added to by the next, etc. This is accomplished by connecting the zinc of one cell to the copper of the next, and the zinc of that to the copper of the third, etc. (Fig. 12.)

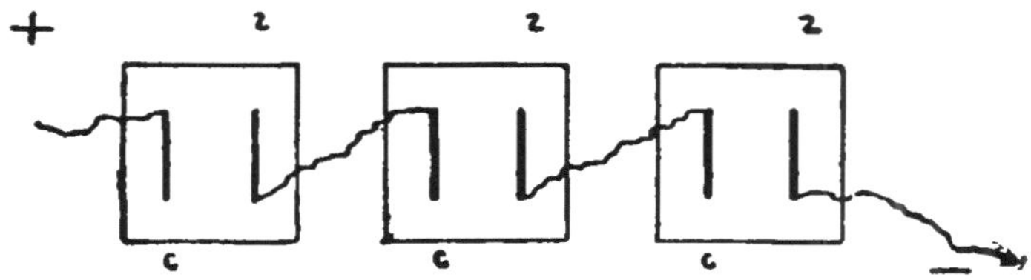

FIG. 12.

This is called a series of cells. The potential of such a series as in the figure would be three times higher than that of a single cell.

When the external resistance is little, not much is gained by increasing the number of cells, as the internal resistance increases in proportion.

Each cell added to the series adds to the current its electro-motive force (E. M. F.), diminished by its internal resistance—the external being of little amount.

Usually the internal resistance, if little, is disregarded and the equation then becomes:

$$C = \frac{E.M.F.}{R}$$

Knowing any two of these fractions we can readily find the third.

$$C = \frac{E.\,M.\,F.}{R},\ \text{or}\ E.M.F. = \frac{C}{R},\ \text{or}\ R = \frac{E.\,M.\,F.}{C}$$

For example—What is the resistance of a conductor through which 12 amperes are passing under a pressure of 60 volts? Ans. $R = 60\frac{E.\,M.\,F.}{12\ C} = 5$ ohms. Or to find the amperes in the following: How many amperes will flow through a conductor having a resistance of 10 ohms under a pressure of 110 volts. Ans. $C=\frac{110 \text{ E. M. F.}}{10 \text{ R}}=11$ amp. How many volts will it take to force 6 amperes through a resistance of one-half ohm? Ans. $\text{E.M.F}=\frac{6 \text{ C}}{\frac{1}{2} \text{ R}}=3$ V.

If now the external resistance is great and we wish to overcome it, we must combine the cells in series as described in Fig. 12. This is also called an intensity battery.

We may also increase the current or value of C. by increasing the size of the plates—if the external resistance is little. This does not increase the electro-motive force (E. M. F.), but lessens the internal resistance, by exposing more plate area to the solution within the cell.

When the resistance is small to overcome, large plates are best, or we can combine all the zinc plates together to form one great zinc cylinder, and all the copper plates together to form a great copper cylinder. This allows of quantity, and the cells so arranged are said to be connected in multiple arc. (See Fig. 13.)

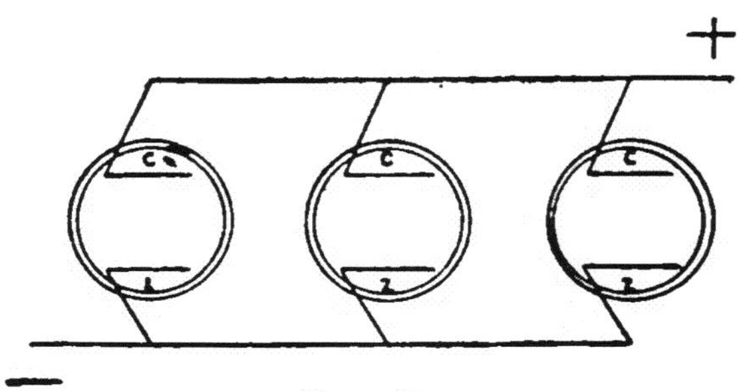

FIG. 13.

Such a battery would be useful where heat is required, as in the cautery. In such a way three times the rate of flow would be obtained than if but one cell were used.

THE WATT.

The energy expended in raising a known weight to a given height is generally taken as a standard for the measurement of work. We adopt the foot pound as a unit of work; by this we mean the amount of work required to raise one pound one foot against the natural force of gravity. If we raise a weight of 30 pounds 3 feet, we have done 90 foot pounds of work, or if we raise 3 pounds to a height of 30 feet, it would be the same.

A horse has the average power to raise 33,000 pounds vertically through one foot of space per minute. Therefore a horse-power is such which can perform 33,000 units of work per minute. The time this work is done in, however, makes a difference. If an engine can do 99,000 units of work in half a minute, it is said to be of three horse-power. Now if a current of electricity can do a certain amount of work, the rate at which such work is done is measured by multiplying the pressure of the current in volts by the amount or rate of flow in amperes, result or product being expressed in watts as the unit of electric power or rate of performing certain electric work.

The watt is equivalent to $\frac{1}{746}$ of a horse-power, as it requires that power to perform 44.25 foot pounds of work per minute, which is $\frac{1}{746}$ of 33,000 foot pounds, which equals one horse-power, or 746 watts to make one electric horse-power (E. H. P.).

If now a dynamo is supplying 30 amperes at a pressure of 50 volts, it must necessarily develop 50 volts multiplied by 30 amperes, or 1,500 watts—or $1\frac{1}{2}$ kilo-watts. If the same dynamo supplies 30 amperes at 50 volts, it is developing the same horse-power as 746 watts is contained times in the product of 30 amperes by 50 volts.

$$30 \times 50 = 1{,}500 \div 746 = 2 + \text{H.P.}$$

THE AMPERE.

The ampere is the unit of the rate of flow of electric current. It is equal to one volt of electro-motive force (E. M. F.) passing through one ohm of resistance. For an example: We again refer to the stream of water going down the mountain side or chute; we have the water chasing downhill, and as it gets to the foot of the hill, or finds its way into the lake or ocean, we note that it has gained rapidity in flowing downward. Say we find the rate of flow at the mouth of the stream at 1,800 gallons per ten hours. Now if you used the water from this stream for a boiler in your factory, and used only as much as would flow into your boiler, which would be filled in one hour, you would use at the rate of 1,800 gallons per ten hours; but during the one hour you have received only 180 gallons in quantity.

If now the electric current flows through the conductor under a pressure of 110 volts, that 110 volts will cause the current to flow at a certain rate, and it is quite evident that a definite quantity has passed in a given time, therefore the ampere is a unit or rate of flow.

THE COULOMB.

If a current of electricity is flowing at the rate of one ampere per second, one coulomb will have passed in that time, designating the quantity of electricity that has passed at the given rate.

THE FARAD.

Capacity of current is measured by a practical unit called the farad. A farad is equal to a coulomb of electricity flowing into a conductor, producing a pressure of one volt.

As the farad is too large a unit to use for our consideration we divide it into micro-farad, signifying the one-millionth of a farad.

CHAPTER III.

BATTERIES AS A SOURCE OF ELECTRICITY.

We may now consider the different forms of primary batteries. A voltaic cell has already been described, the objection to which is that hydrogen accumulates on the copper plates, preventing contact with the liquid and thus obstructing the current.

WE HAVE TWO KINDS OF PRIMARY CELLS.

I. The open circuit. II. The closed circuit cells.

I.

Open circuit cells are adapted to interrupted use and are especially adapted to private houses in connection with bells, annunciators, gas lighting apparatus, etc. The one most generally used and reliable is the Laclanche. The elements are a rod of zinc and a carbon plate surrounded with a layer of peroxide of manganese, to serve as a developing agent. The two elements are placed in a solution of ammonium chloride or sal ammoniac—six ounces to the necessary amount of water.

This is an excellent cell for occasional use, but continuous use wears down the battery and recharging becomes necessary.

The potential of such a cell is about 1.5 volts.

II.

The closed circuit cells are more adapted for constant use, in fact they act better on a normally closed circuit. There are a number of these batteries.

The Daniell cell was the first form of a constant battery made. It is composed of an outer vessel of glass, filled with a saturated solution of sulphate of copper, which, as it is decomposed, is kept saturated by a number of crystals placed at the bottom of the outer jar. A perforated copper cylinder is immersed in the solution, making up the negative element. Inside of this cylinder is placed a thin, porous vessel of earthenware, filled with dilute sulphuric acid (H_2SO_4), in which is placed another cylinder of amalgamated zinc, making up the positive pole of the battery.

The electro-motive force of the Daniell cell is 1.072 volts.

The Bunsen Cell is composed of an outer jar, filled three parts full with a solution of sulphuric acid (H_2SO_4), in which is placed a cylinder of zinc, having a slit at one side for the passage of the liquid. The inner vessel is made of porous earthenware and contains a quantity of nitric acid (H_2NO_3), into which a cylinder of carbon is placed.

These cells when used in great quantities fume considerably, although bichromate of potassium may be substituted for the nitric acid and a saturated solution of chloride of sodium ($NaCl_2$), in place of the acid solution; this however reduces the power considerably.

An excellent battery is that of Grenet—the so-called plunge-battery. It consists of a bottle-shaped glass jar, closed at the top with a hard rubber cap, having two binding posts, mounted upon same, for wire connections. To the inner side of the cap two carbon plates are fastened, reaching almost to the bottom of the jar, and connected at the top with a strip of copper, well varnished to protect it from the fumes or corrosion, to one of the binding posts. In the center of the cap is shown a shoulder of metal with a thumb screw, through the center of which passes a movable brass rod, having a plate of zinc attached to its lower end, encircled by two rubber bands to prevent contact between zinc and carbon. The rod is connected by the aid of a spring to the other binding post. The solution used in this is one of bichromate of potash 10 parts, sulphuric acid (H_2SO_4) 21 parts, and water (H_2O) 69 parts. This is commonly known as Electropion fluid. The solution must always be allowed to cool before using. When freshly made it becomes heated upon mixing the water with the acid, and the latter should be added in small quantities at a time, to avoid a too active chemical reaction.

The battery is immediately set into action by lowering the rod containing the zinc into the liquid, and stopped by raising it above the solution. A number of these connected in series and put into a box, make a very good battery. Electro-motive force (E. M. F.), 1.9 to 2 volts, amperes about 5.

It is best to use the sodium bichromate in place of the bichromate of potash, as the former does not form crystals of chrome alum, which would soon fill up the lower portion of the jar, impeding the action of the elements considerably, and again the sodium is cheaper and much more soluble in water.

The Fuller, another bichromate cell, is one giving a steady current, and can be used at longer intervals than the Grenet cell just described, at about the same electro-motive force (E. M. F.); but the current will only be of three amperes.

A glass jar outside contains a porous earthenware cup, which in turn contains a cone-shaped piece of zinc, attached to a strong copper wire leading upward for connection. Alongside of the porous cup a piece of carbon is placed having at the top a screw or check nut, to facilitate connections. The whole except the carbon is covered with a wooden cover, previously dipped into paraffine, to prevent the creeping upward of the salts contained in the solution, and to avoid corrosion of the brass. It has an opening, allowing the carbon to extend through it, and contains a second opening for the wire from the zinc. The porous cup is filled two-thirds full of a cold solution, composed of sodium chloride ($NaCl_2$) 18 parts and water (H_2O) 72 parts. The electropion fluid used in the Grenet cell is used here within the glass jar, filled about two-thirds full. To facilitate the complete and continuous amalgamation of the zinc, one ounce of metallic mercury is added to the solution in the earthenware cup.

To lessen the internal resistance, is is found advisable to use two or more plates of carbon, connected together outside of the porous cup, so increasing the current considerably, and preventing polarization to a greater extent. Or we can use a large piece of zinc, well amalgamated, and employ a solution of 1 dram of sulphuric acid (H_2SO_4), to the necessary amount of water (H_2O), instead of the sodium chloride.

Throe's solution for the above battery is made as follows: Water 36 parts, potassium bichromate 3 parts, and sulphuric acid (H_2SO_4) 15 parts.

Buttone's solution is made as follows: Chromic acid 6 parts, potassium chromate 1-3 part, sulphuric acid (H_2SO_4) 15 parts, and water (H_2O) 20 parts.

A cheaper modification of the Daniell battery described is the so-called gravity battery, made as follows: At the bottom of a glass jar described is placed a sheet of copper composed of from 4 to 6 pieces of thin sheet copper, set upon their edges in the form of a star; these are united together. A copper wire is attached to this plate, leading upward and out to make up the negative pole. A number of crystals of blue vitriol ($C\ SO_4$), is thrown into the interstices of the copper plate, filling it about to one inch above its base plate. A solution of sulphate of copper is then poured into the jar, covering the star-shaped piece. On top of this is poured a second or weak solution of zinc sulphate to within two inches of the top of the jar. A cast piece of zinc, made in the form of a crow's foot, is lowered into the liquid from the edge of the jar, having a place at its upper extremity for wire connection, making up the positive pole. It will be observed that the two liquids separate, one floating above the other, the copper sulphate remaining at the bottom, whereas the zinc solution remains on top. This is due to the difference in the specific gravity of the two solutions, one being heavier than the other.

The chemical process, when the cell is at work, is an interesting one. The sulphate of copper deposits its metallic salt upon the copper plates and sets free the sulphuric acid (H_2SO_4) so contained, which in turn attacks the zinc upon rising, giving off free sulphate of zinc as a result. As the solution of the copper is denser than the zinc solution, it remains at the bottom.

If the cells are used long in open circuit, the two solutions have a tendency to mix, and the copper will be deposited on the zinc plates, so hindering its action. Or the upper solution of zinc will become saturated, when it will be necessary to remove part of it by decantation, adding water to make up for the amount removed, at the same time throwing in a few handfuls of crystals, which you will find have been gradually used up or decomposed, during the work of the cell. The electro-motive force (E. M. F.) of the cell is one volt, current one-half ampere.

One of the best and later cells made is the Edison-Lalande. They are made in different types, each suitable for a particular kind of work; however, in this class of work, type "S" is most suitable.

The jar is of porcelain and fitted with a porcelain cover from which is suspended a framework of copper, grooved to contain two plates of oxide of copper, the surface of which has been reduced to metallic copper.

The amount of oxide of the plates is so fixed that it will bo entirely reduced to metallic copper, when the zincs are consumed and the solution and battery is exhausted. Two zinc plates are placed on either side of the copper plates, and connected by a machine screw and check nut at the center of the cover, making up the binding post of the zinc element.

The necessary solution is composed of caustic potash (granulated) 2 parts, to water 6 parts, by weight. On top of the solution when cooled is poured 4 ounces of heavy paraffine oil. The latter is used to prevent the creeping of the solution up the zinc, and also to prevent evaporation to a certain extent.

All parts of this battery except the copper frame will have to be renewed when exhausted, as the zincs will be entirely eaten away, and the copper oxide plates reduced to metallic copper.

The solution must always be renewed when the zincs and oxide plates are replaced, as it has become completely saturated with zinc oxide held in solution, and is really changed into zincate of potassium. The solution should always be allowed to cool down before using the battery.

The electro-motive force (E. M. F.) is 0.667 volts, giving a current of 6 amperes—capacity in amperes 300.

We have mentioned amalgamated zincs in the description of batteries. They are prepared by first cleaning the zinc, which should be rolled and not cast so as to render it less porous, then rubbing its surface with a cloth dipped into sulphuric acid, and dropping a few drops of metallic mercury upon the zinc, which is made to expand readily over the entire zinc surface, when rubbed briskly, so subdividing it minutely. The zinc plate will gradually become bright and shiny and ready for use. As the zinc plate or rod is usually attacked at the surface of the acid solution, it is found advisible to protect it by coating its upper end with paraffine wax or heavy shellac varnish.

A COMPARATIVE TABLE OF THE CELLS DESCRIBED.

Name.	E. M. F. Volts.	Int. R. Ohms.	Capacity in Ampere. Hours.	Cont. Cur. Amp.
	V.	O.	A. H.	A.
Laclanche	1.5	0.50	....	....
Daniell..	1.072	0.44	....	.60
Gravity	1.00	0.50	....	.50
Fuller	1.8	0.40	.68	3.00
Grenet	1.9	....	....	5.00
Edison-Lalande	.667	0.025	.300	6.00

CHAPTER IV.

LIGHT AND HEAT EFFECTS OF THE GALVANIC BATTERY.

WE have seen how the phenomena of light and heat can be produced by bringing together the two ends of a wire through which a current flows, and by the spark that is so caused as the current is discharged. If the conducting wires are separated so that a little gap exists between the two, the spark would still try to pass, and in so doing would jump across the space. If two dense pieces of carbon in the form of pencils be connected by wires to the poles of a powerful battery (Fig. 14) in such a way that a current can pass in at the upper piece of carbon and out at the lower piece, are brought in contact as the current is turned on by the aid of a switch, the points of the carbons become immediately incandescent, emitting a light of dazzling brightness. If now the points are slightly separated, the current will still try to pass, but the light between the

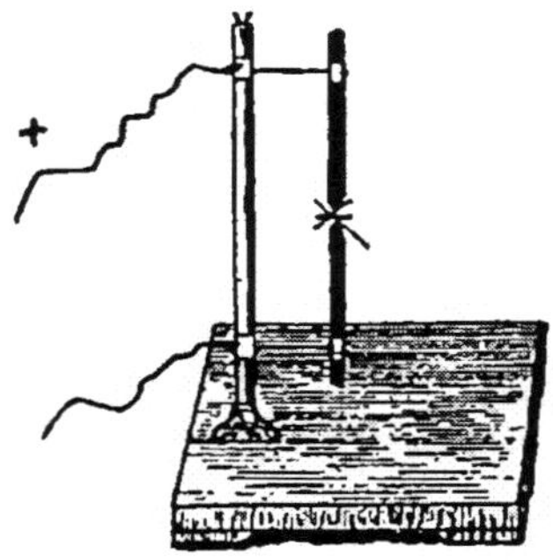

FIG. 14.

ends or points of the carbon is seen to take the form of an arc—called the voltaic arc.

The one or positive carbon point will soon be consumed, whereas the negative one will be added to. From this we conclude that a particle of the positive (+) carbon is to a considerable extent carried over to the negative (—) carbon.

In vacuum this light phenomenon is more manifest. A sort of cone grows upon the negative, and a conical cavity is observed in the positive carbon. As there would be no combustion of the carbon in vacuum, the particles of carbon detached would of course be regularly transferred to the opposite pole.

Another phenomenon is the property of heat, as generated by galvanic electricity, and is demonstrated by the following experiment: Using the same battery as above, we attach to the conductors or wires at their free ends a very fine wire of copper; immediately as the circuit passes, the small wire becomes incandescent, and lastly melts or is dispersed in vapor, burning with brilliancy. This action of heat or incandescence is due to the great resistance offered by the fine wire to the flow of current. The smaller the wire and the less the conducting power of the wire, placed between the conductors, the greater will the resistance to the current be, and the more intense the heat.

On account of the poor conductivity of platinum, offering great resistance to the passage or flow of the current, and becoming red-hot, it has been used successfully for cauterizing tissue in surgical operative treatment.

CHAPTER V.

SECONDARY BATTERIES OR STORAGE CELLS.

IN 1803 Ritter, a German professor of physics,[5] conceived the idea of polarizing metal plates to create a new current; but little or nothing was done for fifty years thereafter, until in 1859, Prof. Gaston Plante discovered that polarization of lead gave stronger phenomena of secondary currents than any other metal, and in 1860 made the first secondary cell.

If a sheet of lead was exposed to the open air for some time, it was discovered to have oxidized or blackened to a certain extent. The oxidized plates were thereupon placed in a jar containing a solution of dilute sulphuric acid, 9 parts water to 1 part acid, and a current of two Bunsen cells was allowed to course through the plates, attaching the positive pole to one plate and the negative to the other. It was immediately observed that the anode, *i.e.*, the plate to which the current from the carbon pole of the battery was attached, became coated with a brown substance, which proved to be peroxide of lead, evidently caused by a chemical reaction going on within the cell, and brought about by the outflowing current, aided by the sulphuric acid.

The opposite plate was deprived of one of its atoms of oxygen which formed upon the anode, reducing the former

5 Wildermann's "Grundlehren der Elektricität," Vol. I., Chap. V., p. 199.

to pure plumbum, or spongy metallic lead, which, as the process went on, became grayish. Finally free hydrogen would be evidenced by the collection of bubbles upon the surface of that plate, which was the signal to discontinue the current going to the cells.

Now by bringing together the free ends of the wires connected to each plate of this secondary cell, a large spark was at once formed and considerable current was perceived; but the current here was found to be reversed from that of the battery current; the positive pole of the battery was found to be negative in the storage cell and the negative pole the positive one; in other words, the charge was the reverse of the discharge.

If the wires of these two charged plates were connected, a current was generated and another chemical action would take place within the cell.

One of the atoms of oxygen of the anode was carried over to the cathode, or spongy metallic lead plate, and combined with it to form monoxide of lead, this would go on until both plates became neutralized or alike, whereupon the secondary battery would be devoid of current and had to be recharged from an outside source.

The accumulating nature of the cell has given it the name of storage cell, for the chemical change of the cell elements caused by a current of another source stored the current.

In reality it is practically the storing of chemical energy.

However, the storage cells of to-day are not so simple in construction as the one of Plante, and the time of the chemical change, which is termed forming, is considerably shortened by the previous use of lead oxides.

The lead plates are cast in the form of grids, which act as supports for the oxides. Molds made of plaster of paris are used for the castings. Pure lead, free of zinc, is used and an odd number of grids have to be made, as the end plates are usually of the same polarity. (Fig. 15.)

The filling of these grids or depressions is called pasting. The positive plate is filled in with a paste composed of litharge and dilute sulphuric acid, one part acid and two parts water.[6]

A wooden spatula will be most suitable for applying the paste. When the grooves are all filled upon one side of the plate, which will then appear smooth, the grid is turned over and treated as the former. It is then set away to dry in a moderately warm place for about 24 hours, and

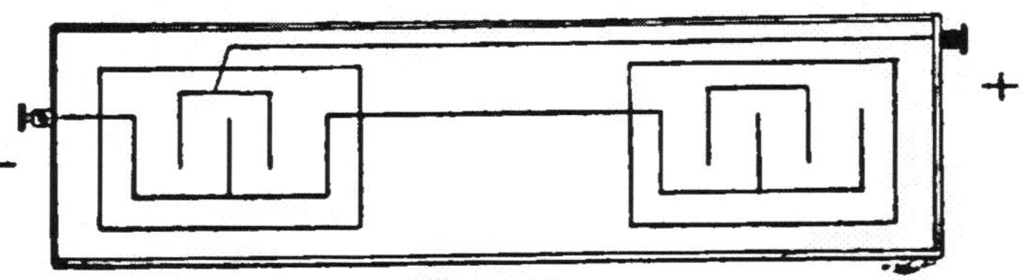

FIG. 15.

placed into a concentrated solution of calcium chloride. which gradually converts the litharge into peroxide of lead.

The negative plates are filled in or pasted in with precipitated lead.

The plates, when ready, are placed alternately into a cell. made of hard rubber or ebonite, using 5 plates in each, 2 positive and 3 negative. The positives are connected together to one conductor and the negatives to another conductor; the cell or cells are put into a transportable case. If more than one is used, the positive pole of cell number one is connected to the negative of number two, and so on.

When this is done, there will be the positive at the one

6 A. E. Livermore, "How to Make an Accumulator, in Practical Radiography," London, p. 17.

end and the negative pole at the other end left open, which, after soldering to the binding posts, become the poles to which the positive and negative leads of the dynamo or battery are to be attached, and the discharging wires to be connected with. The binding posts are led out of the box through holes bored into the case at either end, and are screwed down.

It will be advisable to take a small file and file the figure plus (+) meaning positive and minus (—) meaning negative on the heads of the binding posts, so that the operator or electrician may know one pole from the other in charging or discharging the battery when the box or case is sealed, without having to open it every time it is charged or discharged.

The electrolyte or solution is then put into the cells, composed of pure sulphuric acid 1 part, and water 4 parts, care being taken to add the acid to the water, and not *vice versa.* The solution should cover the top of the plates, the box sealed and a few holes bored in the top for the escape of sulphurous acid gas. It is then ready to be attached to the leads of the dynamo or battery, provided the current be direct and not alternate.

THE CHARGING OF A STORAGE BATTERY.

The charging of such a cell is by no means difficult, but considerable care is necessary, if you have a direct electric current in your office, home or laboratory, or, in other words, a constant potential electric light current. The amount of current necessary depends upon the size of the plates and its composition of elements—for example: We will take a battery with a capacity of 30 amperes. We know what capacity means, and by 30 amperes we mean the delivery of one ampere of current per hour for 30 hours; 2 amperes per hour for 15 hours, etc. It will be necessary to have an ammeter—an instrument for measuring the amperage, and a suitable resistance, which can be provided for as described below, or by a rheostat.

Proceed to charge the storage battery as follows: First, switch off the current to be used, and connect a wire to each wire going to the incandescent lamp, that is, if you take the current from the incandescent light socket. This can be done by wiring up a plug already made for the purpose and which can be purchased from any electric supply dealer at a nominal cost.

If you are puzzled in determining which the positive and negative pole is, you can use Wilke's pole-finding paper[7] as follows: After connecting two wires, the ends of which have been properly bared of their insulating cover, to a screw plug, with the free ends carefully placed a distance apart, screw the plug into the socket and turn on the current by the aid of the switch, then take the Wilke's paper,[8] holding the two wires at either end of it. If a red spot appears upon its surface or end, where it is touched by one of the wires, that spot of color would indicate the negative pole. Now turn off the current and mark the two wires or poles with a lead pencil, or chalk, at the socket for further use.

The resistance or rheostat must now be placed into the circuit. This is an instrument composed of a metal base having a handle on top, to which the negative pole is attached, so constructed to pass over a number of buttons arranged in a semicircle, each indicating a coil composed of German silver wire of known resistance and following one another in connected series, to which the positive pole, which, in this case is the wire coming from the storage battery, is connected.

---

7 A. E. Livermore on "Accumulators in Practical Radiography," London, p. 22.

8 "Description of How to Make Pole Paper," Pharmaceutical Era, March; Scientific American, March 27, 1897.

The handle can be moved from one button or contact piece to the next, backward and forward. The instrument has binding posts mounted upon it for wire connections. One connected with the negative pole of the dynamo or wire, and the positive main leading directly to the positive pole of the battery.

The current or the E. M. F. is varied by the rheostat, by moving the handle as explained, from one contact piece to the other, putting in or taking out the resistance of the little coils of wire, according to the charging rate desired. About 3 amperes per hour is a suitable rate for a 30-hour cell.

The voltage of the source of charge should be about 10 per cent. over that of the battery when fully charged. The potential of a single cell charged varies from 2.4 to 1.7 volts. When the voltage discharge is about 1.8, measured by the volt-meter, the battery should not be used longer, but recharged, as it is not advisable to use up all of the current in a storage cell.

If you cannot obtain a rheostat one may be improvised by filling a porcelain washbowl about half-full of water, then connect the positive wire of the main circuit to a strip of copper 3 inches long and ½ inch wide, bent in such a way that it can be hung upon the edge of the bowl, dipping into the water in the bowl at its lower end. Another piece of copper is connected to a wire at one end, and likewise hung upon the edge of the bowl, leading the other end of the wire to the positive pole of the battery. The two strips of copper should hang directly opposite to each other. From the positive battery pole, lead a wire to the positive pole of the ammeter, and the negative pole of the latter to the socket plug.

Turn on the switch and note the result—there will be a certain amount of current that will pass through the water or resistance, but will hardly move the indicator of the ammeter. If now we permit a drop of sulphuric acid to fall into the bowl, the indicator will at once move forward. This is continued until from 3 to 5 amperes are indicated.

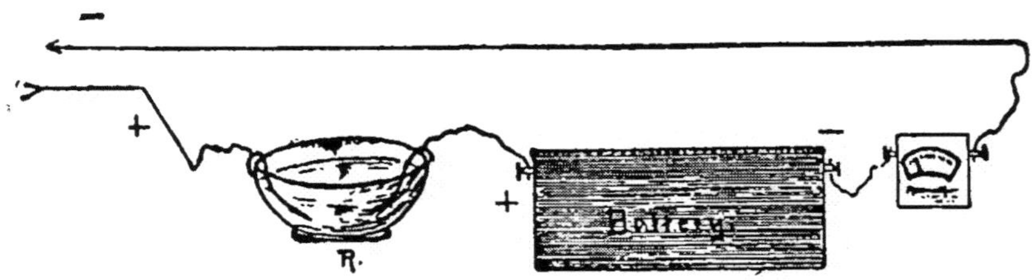

FIG. 16

No more acid is added, and the cells are allowed to charge or fill.

As a substitute for the rheostat, a bank of incandescent lamps connected in multiple series and mounted upon a

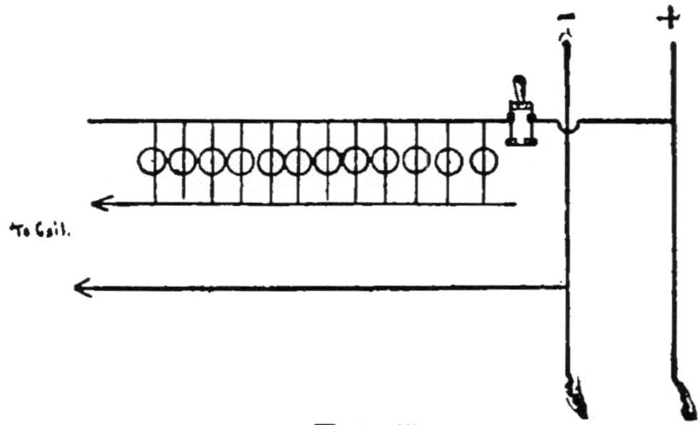

FIG. 17.

suitable board can be used. About twenty 16 c. p. lamps are necessary for a 10 or 12-inch spark coil.

Each 110 volt lamp has a resistance of one-half ohms. If a coil requires 10 amperes, a resistance of 11 ohms will be necessary, stated graphically in the following formula:

$$\text{Current (Amp.)} = \frac{\text{E.M.F.}}{\text{R}} =$$

$$\text{Current in Amp.} = \frac{\text{v. E.M.F}}{\text{11 O. R.}} = \text{10 Amp.}$$

As less resistance or more current is required, one or more lamps may be turned out, or put in. The whole board may be inclosed in a box to shut out the light from the room.

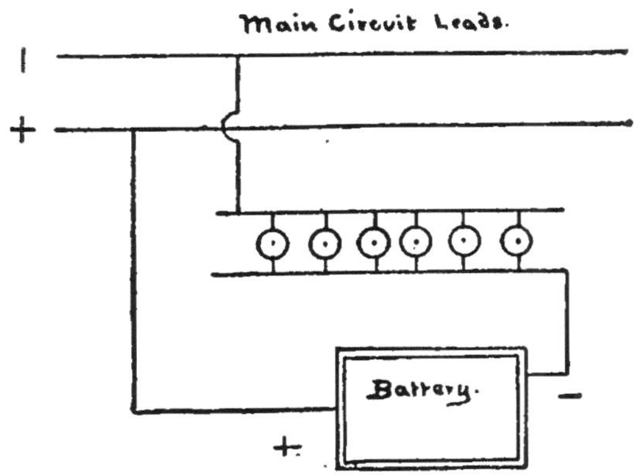

FIG. 1

The cells should charge evenly, one at the same rate as the other, and this charging should be continued until sulphuric acid gas is given off freely from the cells through the little holes made for the purpose, or when the acid solution within the cells takes on a milky appearance.

If now the electro-motive force as represented in volts be measured, by a volt-meter, each cell will indicate about 2.3 volts, if fully charged.

As a certain amount of the liquid in the cell has been lost by evaporation, it should be replaced by the addition of clear water.

Care should be taken in transporting the battery, as it may be injured by jarring, or by displacing the liquid, or breaking the connection between the cells.

CHAPTER VI.

ANIMAL ELECTRICITY.

ALL animal life exhibits, to a certain extent, electrical phenomena ; but few animals can be given here as practically good examples, except the so-called electric-eel and the torpedo-fish. The shock of either of these compares in intensity with that of a powerful leyden jar. The eel is found in the waters of South America and the torpedo-fish in the Mediterranean?[9]

Mattenci showed that sparks would be obtained from such a fish, and that the galvanometer is affected when one wire is held over the body of the fish, and the other placed to the walls of its abdomen. The shock given off is a voluntary one and is undoubtedly used for protection from the attack of enemies, or in killing or maiming its prey for food.

Animal muscular tissue, when contracted, generates a certain amount of electricity. This is more marked in the one than in the other, even when the same muscles are used.

THERMO-ELECTRICITY.

If two bars of dissimilar metals be soldered at their ends in the form of a V (see Fig. 19), and heat is applied at the junction of the two, electricity will be generated, readily detected by connecting the free ends with wires to a galvanometer. The needle of the latter will be immedi-

9 Peck: "Ganot's Physics," p. 507: "Practical Radiography," Snowden, London.

ately deflected as heat is applied—the direction of the current depending upon the metals making up the two, termed or known as a thermo-couple.

If the metal be silver or bismuth, the current will flow from the bismuth to the silver; if iron and German silver are used, the current will flow from silver to iron.

When the heating of the metals is stopped, the current

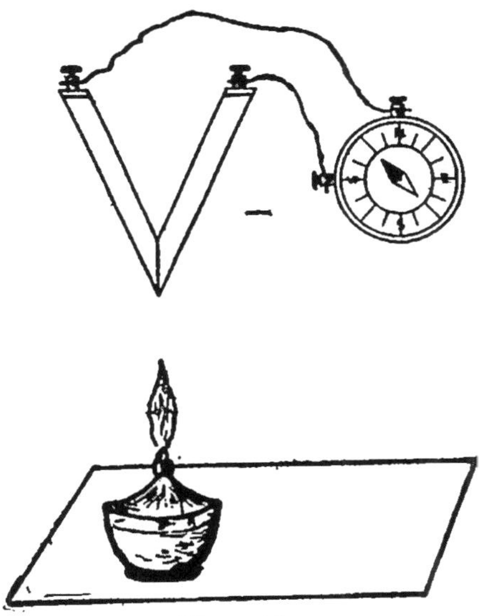

FIG. 19.

will flow in the opposite direction—as again indicated by the magnetic needle—until both metals are of even or equal temperature, when it will resume its natural meridian.

If a number of these couples be joined, they form a thermo-electric pile or battery.

In this way we can get a more powerful current than in the single couple, by heating as above.

The cause of electricity in this example is due to the unequal heating of two unlike metals.

PYRO-ELECTRICITY.

Many crystals, when heated, exhibit opposite electricity at their opposite ends.

The extremity of a pole of a crystal which is positive while heated, will become negative when the temperature falls. The result is entirely one of heat, and is never shown by crystals at their constant temperatures.

The pyro-electrical effect was first observed in tourmaline,[10] which was found to possess the property of attracting light bodies to it when heated, and repelling them when cold.

The phenomena is also shown in zinc silicate, or electric calamine, boracite, Brazilian topaz, and many others.

PLANT ELECTRICITY.

The *Phytolacca electrica*, a Brazilian plant, said to have been lately discovered, is said to have certain electrical properties, and the charge or shock given off by same is claimed to be about equal to one Daniell cell.

---

10 Watts' "Physical Chemistry," Fowne.

CHAPTER VII.

MAGNETO INDUCED ELECTRICITY OR ELECTRO-DYNAMICS.

We have described how Orsted, of Copenhagen, in 1819, observed an intimate relation between magnetism and electricity, and how he discovered the galvanoscope, and that his theory was fully developed by Ampère.

We have seen how a bar of soft iron, bent in the form of a horseshoe, can be made a magnet, by winding a coil of insulated wire around it in the form of a solenoid and allowing a current from a battery to flow through the latter. It has also been shown by the example of the phenomena of momentary currents (Fig. 8) caused by passing a permanent bar magnet into the helix of a solenoid connected to a galvanometer, and how these momentary currents deflected the needle—first one way and then the other as the magnet is presented to it or withdrawn.

It has been fully described how the helix of the coil as well as the bar became magnetized.

Faraday's experiment is demonstrated as follows: Take two bobbins of wood, one made to fit inside of the other, and wind over each a few layers of silk-covered insulated copper wire. We have two coils, the smaller or inner one we will name the primary, as its terminals are connected with the poles of a battery or cell, and the outer coil, or larger one, the secondary. If connected as shown in the illustration, and the smaller coil be introduced into the larger one, a deflection of the needle in one direction will at once be observed—the needle gradually settling back to its neutral point. If the current flowing to the primary coil is stopped by cutting or disconnecting the wires, another current will be produced which is also momentary, but in the opposite direction, returning to its neutral point after a few wild oscillations. (Fig. 20.)

These momentary actions are named Induced Current Phenomena. The current going to the galvanometer is said to be an induced or secondary current. If the primary current be an interrupted one, brought about by rapidly connecting and disconnecting the cut ends of the wires

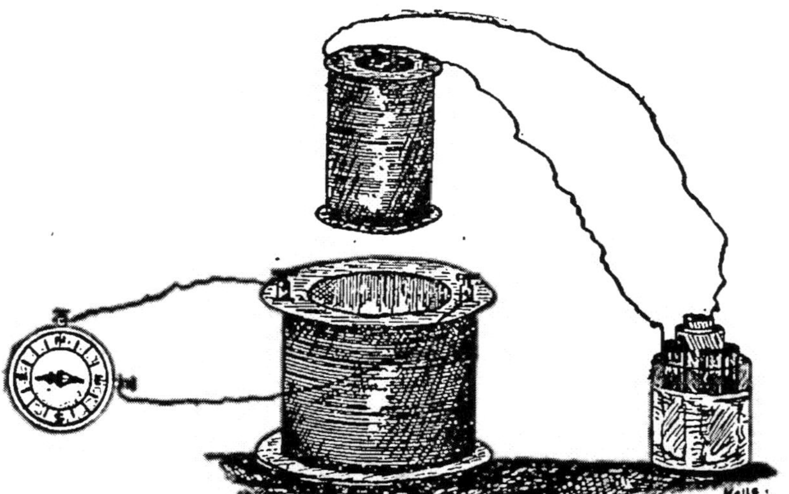

FIG. 20.

from the battery, we have the needle sway to and fro from either side of its neutral line or meridian, within a certain space or degrees, marked upon the tangent.

If, instead of the interruption of the primary current, we increase and decrease the current of the battery, the same effect upon the needle is produced.

The following are the laws of induced currents:

I. At the instant when the primary current begins to flow or to increase its intensity, an induced current, inverse and momentary, is developed in the secondary coil or circuit.

II. The primary current approaching the conductor gives rise to an induced current in the secondary coil inverse and momentary.

III. At the moment this current ceases, or when its intensity diminishes, or when it is reversed from an adjacent coil, an induced current begins with the secondary coil or circuit, direct and momentary.

We can see how light and heat could be produced by the galvanic battery current, but can also readily imagine that the production of enough light to illuminate an ordinary dwelling would involve a great expense and labor to keep the batteries in running order, by introducing new zincs, carbons and solutions. Thousands of cells would perhaps be necessary.

Now consider the number of cells and the cost of lighting one of New York City's 24-story buildings, at the same time furnishing power to run the passenger elevators and perhaps printing presses in the basement. When we consider these facts it will be readily seen how vastly economical the making of a fire is, and replenishing the fire with coal, to produce steam, which can be utilized in generating electricity.

In the generation of current we have the discovery of Michael Faraday, an English scientist, who properly applied the so-called Volta induction to electro-dynamics in 1831, and upon whose principle the great generators of the present day are built, furnishing thousands, even millions of buildings, with light and power. The details pertaining to the principles of induction, relating to their value in radiography, will be described in Part II., Chapter I.

There are two general classes of these generating dynamical electrical machines, named after the kind of currents generated or delivered by each. They are (1) a continuous or direct current generator and (2) the alternating current generator.

As it will be important in the future to refer to these machines, it is deemed advisable to give a short outline and description of each.

I.

THE CONTINUOUS CURRENT DYNAMO.

The first so-called magnetic electric machine was made by Professor Pixii, September 30, 1832—about a year after the discovery of Faraday, and publicly demonstrated in Paris at that time.[11]

It consisted of an armature made with two pole projections upon which were wound a coil of insulated wire.

The permanent horseshoe magnet was made to rotate rapidly in front of the faces of the armature, so that the induced polarity could be rapidly reversed. Electromagnetic currents would be produced in the armature, which in turn were carried to the coils of wire by induction and thence outward.

Clarke, in 1834, made another form of machine wherein the armature, containing the coils of wire, rotated inside of the magnet as in Pixii's.

In 1835, Page made one in which both magnet and coils were stationary, and the armature of soft iron alone was made to rotate.

Stöhrer, a German scientist, made the first practical dynamo-electric machine, wherein a number of the coils,

11 Wildermann, "Grundlehre der Elektricität," s. 145.

wound collectively upon one armature, were made to rotate before the faces of several magnetic poles.

The practical points here are the same as in the Pixii machine, except in the change of form; however, one difference is observed in the figure, and that is, at the upper extremity there is a shoulder cap, having a division or fissure on each side, like the section of a split tube. This is called the commutator, receiving on one side one wire of the induction coil, and on the other half the other wire.

The springs, instead of being placed on either side, are here one above the other, and called brushes or collectors.

The use of this commutator or split tube arrangement is to deliver a continuous or direct current in one direction only, accomplished by the first brush pressing upon one-

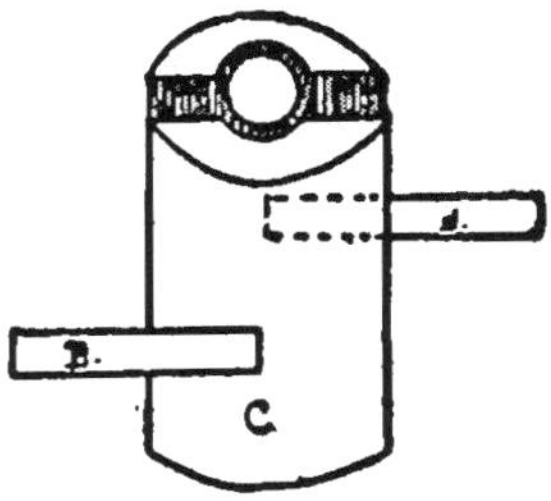

FIG. 21.

half of the commutator to which one wire of the coil is connected, receiving the momentary or induced current, and that, by turning the shaft, the other half of the commutator or tube to which the other wire of the coil is connected, comes in contact with the lower spring or brush and another induced current is received, although the two halves receive an alternate momentary current, brought about by the rapid revolution of the commutator or split tube arrangement rapidly changing its positive and negative halves. (Fig. 21.)

The brushes are stationary and serve to collect the current at the positive and negative poles. The continuous current is most suitable for electric incandescent lighting or motor work, whereas the alternating current dynamo is better adapted to arc or street lighting.

II.

ALTERNATING CURRENT DYNAMOS.

If we replace the split tube arrangement of the small continuous dynamo, just described, by mounting two entire rings upon the shaft where the commutator has been, and connect one wire of the coils of the armature to one ring, and the other wire to the other ring, and place the brushes or springs in contact with each ring, we need only to turn the shaft when an entirely different current will be delivered.

Instead of an even current in one direction as given off by the machine previously described, we will experience a number of to and fro currents—practically a delivery of the first original momentary induced current that Ampère noticed in the experiments described.

This dynamo is called an alternating dynamo on account of the kind of current it delivers to the external curcuit. This class of dynamo is best adapted to arc lighting, but can be used for radiography, as will be later described.

DYNAMO COMPONENTS.

The magnets of dynamos of the present day are not permanent, but are electro-magnets, made of wrought iron, except that part called the pole pieces, which are cast iron and constituting the north and south poles in which the armature revolves. (Fig. 22.)

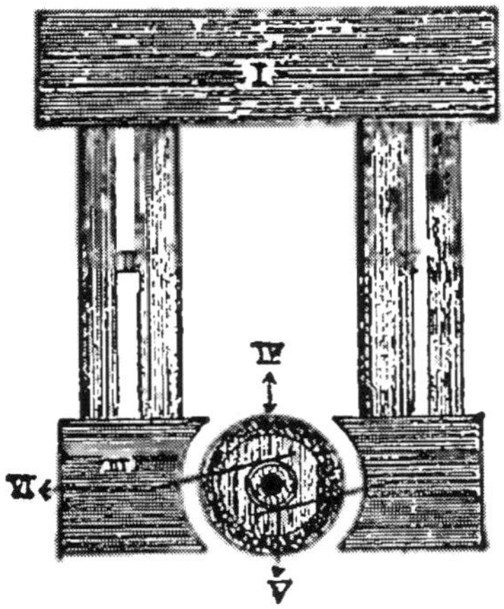

I. Magnetic Yoke.
II. Cores.
III. Pole Pieces.
IV. Armature.
V. Commutator.
VI. Brushes.

FIG. 22.

The yoke at the top joins the cores on either side, over which are wound the coils of wire necessary to make the whole an electric magnet.

PART II.

The Practical and Theoretical Advance and Application of Radiography.

PART II.

CHAPTER I.

As early as 1831 Professor Faraday,[12] the so-called "Father of Disruptive Currents," demonstrated his discovery of the secondary or induced currents by using two iron rings, placed one inside of the other, upon which were wound two coils of copper wire, well insulated from each other and the rings or cores. The one coil which we will call the primary—inasmuch as it was connected in circuit with a battery of 10 cells; and the other the secondary, the terminals of which were connected to a magnetometer.

By disconnecting one of the wires leading from the battery to the primary coil, the needle would be wildly deflected, and by bringing the ends of the wire together the needle would be deflected in an opposite direction.

Faraday did not then, however, discover the fact, that the secondary or induced current was transformed to a much higher E. M. F. than that of the primary battery current.

Later, it was found that this secondary or induced current was greatly increased by rapidly connecting and disconnecting one pole or wire leading from the battery to the primary coil.

This was demonstrated by rubbing the rough surface of a file, connected at one end to a wire leading to the battery, with the other or free terminals coming from the battery;

---

12 "Experimental Researches," Proc. Royal Soc., 1841.

in other words, the file becomes the one pole, and the free wire which was to be used to run over the rough surface of the former becomes the other.

By rapidly passing the free wire end up and down the ribbed surface, sparks would rapidly pass between the free ends of the secondary coil at a much greater distance than when the primary circuit was merely made and broken.

The file was replaced later by an automatic device termed Rheotome, as will be minutely described in Chapter III. It is an automatic arrangement, made to produce a rapid

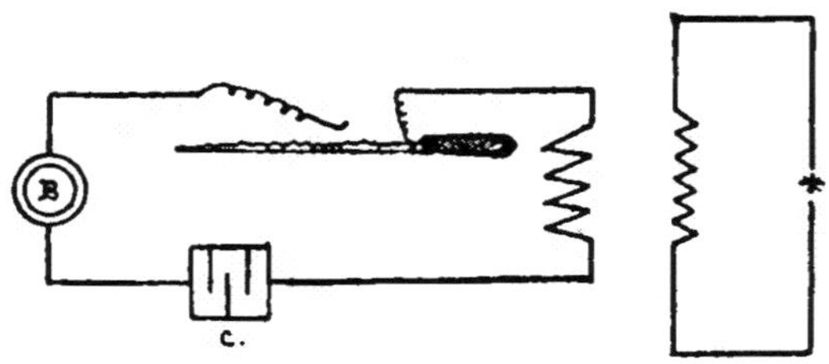

FIG. 23

charge and discharge of the initial current through the primary coil when connected to the battery.

Condensers are accumulators of current, and are made of an insulated body between two metallic layers; formerly made in the form of a leyden jar, or by cementing two sheets of tin foil to glass plates and connecting the tin foil sheets alternately to the positive and negative poles in circuit with the primary current.

Instead of the glass plates, paraffine paper is now used. By connecting this condenser, in the way described, to the terminals of the make-and-brake arrangement, Rheotome or circuit breaker of the primary current, Professor Fizeau[13] found it would greatly increase the secondary current and its spark, and also that the spark at the Rheotome was considerably diminished.

13 Pynchon, p. 456.

By rubbing the wire over the file (Fig. 23), considerable sparking resulted, which by the use of a condenser was obviated, as all of the overcharge, as it were, was stored by the condenser, to be dealt out to the secondary coil, by induction, as it was used up at its poles or terminals.

The use of the circuit breaker and condenser will be described in Chapter III., so that we will pass on to the uses of the induced secondary or disruptive spark discharge.

The spark discharge, when mentioned, refers to that

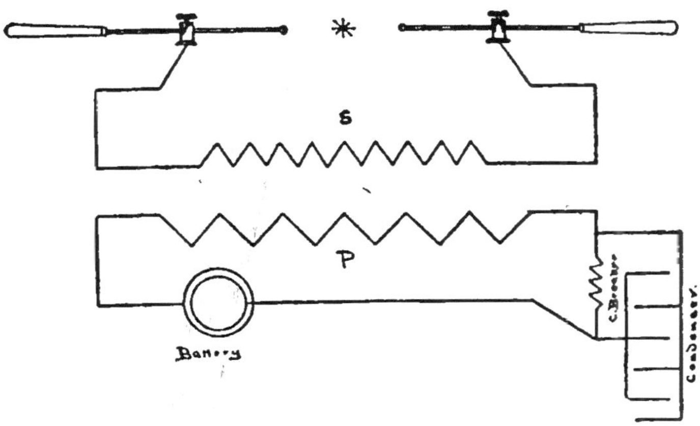

FIG. 24.

phenomena passing between the positive and negative poles of the secondary coil.

The poles as shown in the figure are separated, leaving a space between for the spark to pass, which is termed the spark gap.

By closely studying Fig. 24 you may readily trace the current from the battery to the circuit breaker, to condenser, to primary coil; then observe a space, corresponding to the insulated portion between the two coils, primary (P) and secondary (S). The terminals or poles of the latter ending in wires containing small metallic balls at their inner end, and wooden handles at their outer ends, to facilitate separating them from one another, leaving the space between, known as the spark gap.

Faraday noticed that when the secondary poles were brought very near together, the spark would become more and more active, and lastly melt the metal of the pole ends; and furthermore that the loud crackling sound became higher in pitch by using smaller ball terminals, varying with their size in the pitch and tone produced.[14]

He also found that by allowing the spark to pass through rarified air, the color of the spark would change from purple, as in ordinary atmosphere, to a purple rose, etc. He used a number of different gases in such a way, all giving the spark a distinct color.

He divided electrical effect or discharge into several modes.

1. That of simple conduction, involving no change or displacement of particles.

2. Electrical discharge, with the display to a certain degree of the particles concerned.

3. The mode of sparking or brushes, because of the violent displacement of the particles of the dielectrics in its course, may be called disruptive discharge.

4. This mode may be distinguished by the words convection or carrying discharge, being that in which discharge is effected either by carrying power of solid particles or those of gases or liquids.

Later, Maxwell,[15] his assistant, combined the three first modes in one, and argued that luminiferous ether was the medium of transmission of electricity, light, and magnetism.

Interesting experiments showed that the sparks would penetrate cardboard and even glass. When placed between

---

14 Phil. Trans., 1837.

15 "Treatise on Electricity and Magnetism," Vol. I.

the spark terminals, a plate of glass almost six inches thick was pierced by sparks from a very large induction apparatus.[16]

The duration of the spark was demonstrated by Wheatestone,[17] who used a rotating field of glass sections of various colors. By looking at the rapidity of the rotated field in reflected sunlight, the colors would be found to blend into a neutral tint, but when a spark was allowed to pass in front of it, the various colors could be readily distinguished by the eye. He claimed the duration of a spark to be .000042th of a second.

You can readily see how many scientists must have experimented with this secondary current, as it was then a new discovery and hundreds of experiments are recorded. However, those most interesting were the experiments made in passing or discharging the spark in rarified gas or atmosphere. The latter led to the making of numberless tubes and globes of glass, containing electrodes of various metals, and exhausting the air or gas within the tubes, by the use of mechanical air pumps.

The first tubes were made by Geissler,[18] in 1858 to 1859. They were made of glass containing platinum electrodes, fused into the glass at opposite ends. He observed the peculiar phenomenon within such a tube, when connected in circuit with a battery of 500 cells. He also showed that by rubbing the tube when cold, with an insulated body, such as silk, a certain glow was produced, and that its color would vary with the kind or amount of residual gas within the tube.[19]

De La Rue and Miller [20] in 1877 used a powerful battery of

---

16 Encyclopedia Britannica, "Electricity."

17 Phil. Trans., 1834.

18 Encyclo. Brit., vol. viii., p. 64. Pogg., Annal., 1858–59.

19 Science Record, 1873.

20 Wildermann, Grundl. der Elek., p. 46.

8,040 chloride cells in connection with a vacuum tube, and found that the discharge within the same was disruptive—assuming the same nature as that displayed in the open atmosphere.

In 1825 Morgan[21] demonstrated that an electric discharge would not pass through a perfect vacuum, in other words, if the tube was exhausted of every particle of air within it, and connected to the terminals of an electric machine, no luminosity was observed—the current, instead of producing the light within the tube, crossed in sparks over the exterior of the bulb to its opposite pole. Therefore the highest possible vacuum acts as a dielectric.

Professor Hittorf,[22] in 1859 to 1860, found that by applying a magnet to the outside of a glass vacuum tube, while in circuit, he was enabled to deflect or draw toward the magnet the stream of luminosity, and that the light would follow the magnetic lines and could be drawn toward the side of the tube nearest to the poles of the magnet.

Later we come to the novel discovery by Professor Gassiot. We have noted the discoveries of the various scientists, and are told of the peculiar glow as shown within exhausted tubes, when connected to a battery of numerous cells. Here then is Gassiot using 1,080 chloride of silver cells connected in series—imagine for a moment; nearly 2,000 of these cells giving about 2,000 volts connected to a small tube, and so very much depending upon the result, as we shall learn.

It was found by using the battery, in connection with the ordinary tin foil condenser, connected to the tube, that not only did the luminosity appear within the tube, but that the light phenomena was divided into layers or striæ, so called, resembling somewhat the striæ of voluntary muscle fiber as seen under the miscroscope—a light area, and then a dark

---

21 Wiedemann, Annalen, vol. ii.; Phil. Trans., 1875, vol. lxxv.

22 Pogg., Annalen, 1858 to 1869; Ganot's Phys., p. 925.

one, originating at the negative pole or cathode and streaming toward the positive or anode.[23]

This led to another investigation, and Spottiswoode, the assistant to Gassiot, determined that these striæ must be due to the vibrations of the current. They applied a vacuum tube, during one of their experiments, to the secondary terminals of the induction apparatus, and again the tube was filled with light.

It is true that Geissler made the first vacuum tube, but his tubes were all of low vacuum, about .0025 degrees and filled with the various gases, making excellent material for demonstrations, owing to their peculiarity in forming colors, *i.e.*, carbonic acid gas gave an opalescent-green tint, nitrogen an orange yellow, hydrogen a white and red color, etc. But it was Professor Crookes, who first ascertained the proper vacuum for these tubes, and designated for disruptive currents.

The tubes, as made by Crookes, were exhausted by the use of the Geissler[24] air pump and a chemical air-drying process. He claims to have produced, in this way, a vacuum within a tube of .000001th degree of atmospheric pressure —equal to a barometric column of mercury three miles high.

Upon allowing a disruptive discharge of high electromotive force coming from the poles of the secondary coil of an induction apparatus, to course through such a tube, he observed the same luminosity within it as described.

This light phenomena or radiation he credited to the molecular bombardment of the rarified gas particles, put into motion by the electric discharge. He claimed that

23 Proc. Roy. Soc., vol. x., pp. 36, 393, 404; xii., p. 329; xxiii., p. 356.

24 Norrie: "Currents in Vacuo," p. 94; Crookes' Lect. Brit. Asso., Sheffield, Eng., Aug. 22, 1879.

the individual gas particles were enormously subdivided, and violently thrown against each other in the vain attempt to escape from the tube, and that through this wild motion or bombardment the light was caused.[25]

A very peculiar fact noted, was that the light did not commence directly at the negative pole, but that a dark area (*Dunkle schicht*)[26] encircled that pole, using a tube with platinum terminals, as positive and negative, at the opposite ends.

Crookes found that by using both ends as the positive electrode and a negative electrode composed of a fine strip of platinum, placed in the center of the tube, the following results were observed : a dark area on either side of the negative and bright light at the positive poles.

From this he deduced that the gas particles were first set in motion at the negative pole, and traveled in straight lines forward, meeting the resistance of the returning particles at the space where the light appeared.

If the vacuum was increased, the dark area would be greater, owing to the still greater rarity of the particles of gas within the tube traveling a greater distance without the disturbance or rebombardment of the returning ones.

It became quite evident to him that, as there had been heretofore only three forms or states of matter—namely, solids, liquids, and gases, that in the case with the tube, a fourth must exist in the form of radiance. Therefore he added the ultra-gaseous or radiant state.

This radiant state was observed. as said, in rarified air or vacuum of high degree as described. The ray matter in the case of ordinary air—that is, where no gas had been

25 Crookes' Roy. Inst. Proc., April 4, 1879, vol. lx., p. 138; Roy. Soc. Trans., 1874; Lord Kelvin, Address Roy. Soc., Nov., 1893; The Elect., London, Feb. 14, 1896.

26 Gordon: "A Physical Treatise on Electricity and Magnetism," Crookes' Lect. Brit. Asso., Sheffield, Eng., Aug. 22, 1879.

introduced into the tubes, was found to be of a peculiar violet or ultra-violet color, coming in streams or straight

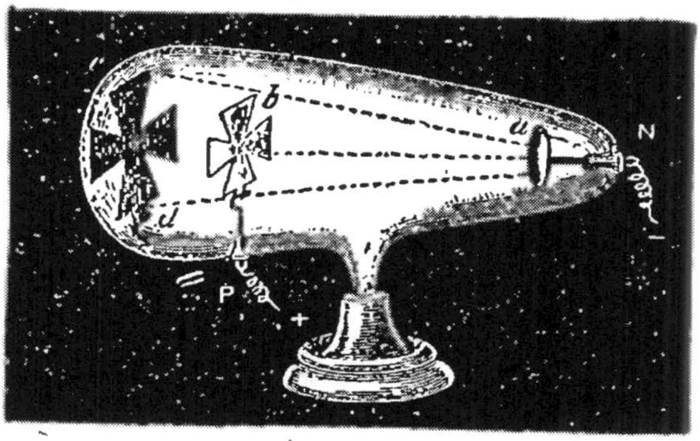

FIG. 25.

lines from the negative pole. He therefore termed them cathode rays. When the vacuum was very high, *i.e.*,

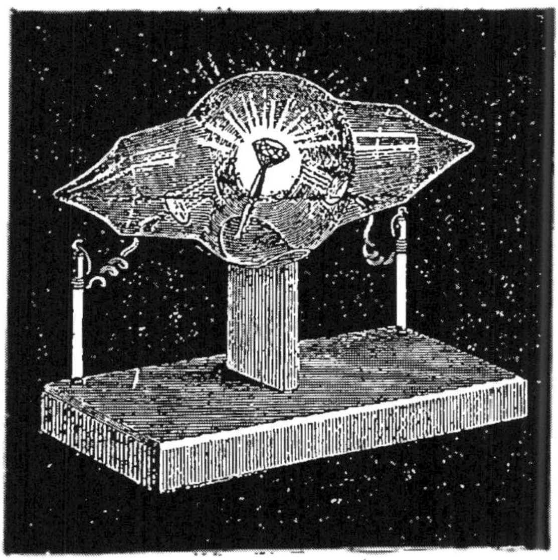

FIG. 26.

.0000001, there was naturally a scarcity of the air particles, and therefore the dark area had to be greater, whereas the end of the tube opposite the negative had to increase in brightness.

He introduced a maltese cross inside of the tube (Fig. 25), and a dark area or shadow of the exact image appeared upon the side of the globe—thus proving the molecular bombardment theory. The highly vibrated molecules would strike the metal cross, and, being unable to pierce it, would be thrown back toward the negative pole, whereas the uninterrupted particles continued in straight lines and only met opposition at the end of the tube, or its walls.

By introducing precious stones into the tube, *i.e.*, a

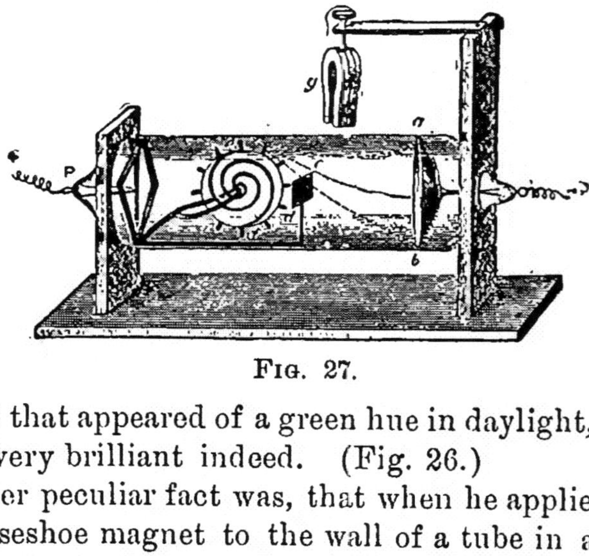

FIG. 27.

diamond that appeared of a green hue in daylight, the stone became very brilliant indeed. (Fig. 26.)

Another peculiar fact was, that when he applied an ordinary horseshoe magnet to the wall of a tube in action the ray of light would immediately be deflected toward that side.

To demonstrate this fact and the bombardment theory, he had a very ingenious tube constructed, containing a waterwheel at the positive end of the tube. By applying a magnet at one side the wheel would be made to revolve rapidly in the opposite direction. If the magnet was then held on the other side, directly opposite where it had been placed at first, the wheel would revolve reversely. (Fig. 27.)

So much, then, for the Crookes tube, and the fourth

state of matter. It might be mentioned that through these experiments Professor Crookes discovered the radiometer, such as are exhibited in the windows of opticians, etc., consisting of a bulb of glass containing four platinum foil vanes blackened upon one side and adjusted to a common shaft. They are made to revolve when exposed to the rays of sunlight.

The reader will now understand what is meant by the cathode ray, as that term may be conflicted with the X rays hereinafter described. By making the negative in the form of a concave mirror the stream of light could be concentrated into a spot upon the opposite end of the tube, and, while in action, the glass in the neighborhood of this spot of fluorescence will become quite hot; in fact, sealing-wax can be melted at this point, and if the discharge is kept up still longer the glass will crack; the vacuum will remain, however, until the electrical action is carried still further. Then the glass will become soft, and the pressure of the air without will be forced through, entering the tube and ruining the vacuum.

Crookes heated and even melted pieces of metal wire (irido-platinum) within these tubes.

For a number of years nothing was accomplished with this cathode ray until, in 1892, Professor Herz[27] discovered that these cathode rays—as he thought them to be—would penetrate gold leaf. He accomplished this by covering a small piece of uranium or Anna glass with gold leaf, leaving an uncovered edge of glass exposed all around. By bringing this piece of glass near the tube and opposite the cathode pole he found that the piece of glass which was uncovered became fluorescent, and that if he increased the vacuum still more within the tube even the glass in the back of the leaf was rendered fluorescent.

He then tried a number of other substances, such as

27 Wiedemann's "Annalen," N. P. 45, 28, 1892.

zinc, carbon, aluminium, tin foil, etc. Aluminium allowed the rays to pass very freely.

The early death of this great scientist threw the matter into his assistant's hands, who closely followed the advanced ideas of his predecessor. This was Professor Lenard, and he came nearest to the finding of the X rays.[28] He found that the cathode rays not only existed inside of the tube, but that they also passed through the walls, and showed certain properties in open air.

For this experiment, a tube having an aluminium window, as he called it, was made and connected to a vacuum pump, so that the pressure of .00002 mm. within could be increased or decreased at will. The window in this tube consisted of an aluminium disk glued to a metal cap having a perforation at its center, corresponding to the aluminium

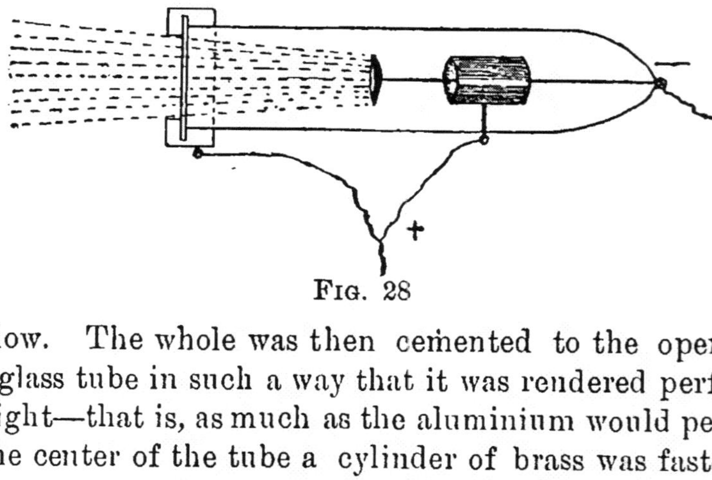

FIG. 28

window. The whole was then cemented to the open end of a glass tube in such a way that it was rendered perfectly air-tight—that is, as much as the aluminium would permit. In the center of the tube a cylinder of brass was fastened. The cap containing the window and the latter were connected to the anode pole.

The cathode pole consisted of a platinum wire and a disk, reaching from the end of the tube beyond and through the cylinder of the anode. (Fig. 28.)

28 Wiedemann's "Annalen," vol. lvi., p. 225; Lenard, "The Elect.," London, March 23, 30, 1894; Lenard, "The Elect.," London, April 6, 1894; Lenard, "Elect. Review," London, January 24, 1896.

When the current was turned into such a tube the cathode stream of light would be thrown forward toward the window, and by looking closely a faint violet light would be observed near that end of the tube, disappearing at a distance of 4½ inches.

If such substances as become fluorescent or phosphorescent within the tube, or in sunlight, were exposed to the rays emitted from this tube, fluorescence outside and beyond the distance described was obtained.

Lenard experimented with a number of chemicals and found that the barium and potassium cyanides of platinum, different kinds of glass, such as flint, uranium, etc., sulphide of quinine in powder form, etc., and found them more or less fluorescent.

If tin foil or thin glass were interposed between the end of the tube and a screen containing one of the above chemicals, the phosphorescence was not so marked. A screen made of a piece of paper and coated with fused pentadecylparatolylcetone he found to be highly fluorescent.

The light without the tube was discovered to penetrate gold and silver leaf, tissue paper, writing paper, and thin cardboard to a certain extent, while all cast a shadow upon the screen mentioned. A drop of water appeared as a black shadow.

Lenard must have been puzzled at all these phenomena. Aluminium, or even tin foil, when placed within the tube, cast a shadow; whereas, here it was pierced almost entirely; undoubtedly he was dealing with very weak X rays.

He substituted the aluminium window of the former tube by closing the opening with very thin glass, and again observed the same phenomena. All this did not convince him that there must be a difference in the two kinds of rays, but he firmly believed them to be cathode, and referred to the experiments of Crookes as being handicapped by not having the proper vacuum in his tubes, or that the cathode rays in Crookes' experiments differed from those found by him.

Not satisfied with these facts, he resorted to the sensitive photographic bromide or silver paper, and found that if brought near the aluminium window it became slightly clouded or blackened—perhaps equal to an outdoor exposure to fogged sunlight.

By using photographic plates he obtained, upon developing, a permanent record of the penetrating property of this ray. A plate covered partly with aluminium was darkened some, but not as much as when the metal had not been used.

Quartz was found to give lighter shading than aluminium, comparing the positive images.

A novel picture was made by laying strips of metal upon cardboard placed in contact with the film of the photographic plate and exposed to the rays. The plate, when developed, showed the light lines corresponding to the metals, and dark lines where the cardboard had been—(Negative image).

Charged bodies, consisting of metallic plates, were found to be discharged when brought within the ray emanations outside of the tube, when either positively or negatively charged, and rapidly rendered free of any electric properties, even at a much greater distance than that which caused fluorescence of the screen.

Lenard strongly retained the belief of Crookes and his theory as substantiated by Hertz and perhaps scores of other scientists.

De Kowalski used a tube having no electrodes[29] fused into its walls. By placing the tube near to the poles of a discharger—using the Tesla transformer described later—obtained cathode rays. He even obtained results similar

29 DeKowalski, Acad. Sci., Paris, Jan. 14, 1895; Soc. Franc. Phys., January, 1895; Nature, London, Jan. 24, 1895; Feb. 21, 1895.

to that of Roentgen, but alas! did not see into the mystery of the cathode and an independent ray.

After all these years of experimental research, it remained for Prof. William K. Roentgen, professor of physics in the Pleicher Ring Laboratory of the Royal University of Wurzburg, to discover the value of the vacuum tube and the phenomena of another kind of rays.

The collective properties of the cathode rays, up to the time of his discovery, may be given in the following tabulated form:

1. The cathode rays were observed in high vacuo.
2. They proceed from the cathode or negative pole.
3. That the stream is composed of molecules or particles streaming in straight lines from the cathode.
4. That the bombardment of the vibrated electrofied particles within caused fluorescence of the glass walls of the tube.
5. That this bombardment against the walls of the glass tube caused fluorescence of the tube itself or chemical bodies included within the tube.
6. That this cathode stream can be deflected from its straight course by a magnet applied externally to the tube wall.
7. That the rays are concentrated by a concave disk, causing a fluorescent spot.
8. That the rays exhibited heat properties, as shown by the concentrated ray, heating the glass, melting wax, softening glass, and even melting irrido-platinum wire.

On November 8,1895, Professor Roentgen,[30] while experimenting with a Crookes' tube covered with black cardboard perfectly impervious to light, found that a piece of paper coated with barium-platino-cyanide became highly fluorescent.

---

30 Roentgen: Wurz. Physik. Med. Gesell., January, 1895; Nature, London, January, 1896; Elect., London, April 24, 1896; Sitz. Wurz. Physik. Inst., March 9, 1896.

He knew that this change must be due to light from some source. No light could come from the tube, as that was covered with black cardboard, which was not only impervious but would not even transmit the strongest light known.

Investigation confirmed the fact, however, that the light came from the covered tube and that he was dealing with a heretofore undescribed electro-physical force, although having a power resembling somewhat that of the ultra-violet rays of the solar spectrum and the cathode rays of Crookes, Herz, and Lenard.

CHAPTER II.

A NEW FORM OF RADIATION.[31]

BY PROF. WILHELM KONRAD ROENTGEN.

(1) If we pass the discharge from a large Ruhmkorff coil through a Hittorf or a sufficiently exhausted Lenard, Crookes, or similar tubes, and cover it with a somewhat closely-fitted mantle of thin black cardboard, we observe in a completely darkened room that a paper screen, washed with barium-platino-cyanide, lights up brilliantly and fluoresces equally well whether the treated side or the other be turned toward the discharge tube. Fluorescence is still observable two meters away from the apparatus. It is easy to convince oneself that the cause of the fluorescence is the discharge apparatus and nothing else.

(2) The most striking feature of this phenomenon is that an influence (*agens*) capable of exciting brilliant fluorescence is able to pass through the black cardboard cover, which transmits none of the ultra-violet rays of the sun or of the electric arc, and one immediately inquires whether other bodies possess this property. It is soon discovered that all bodies are transparent to this influence, but in very different degrees. A few examples will suffice.

Paper is very transparent; the fluorescent screen held behind a bound volume of 1,000 pages lighted up brightly; the printer's ink offered no perceptible obstacle. Fluorescence was also noted behind two packs of cards; a few

31 Preliminary communication to the Wurzburg Physico-Medical Society, December, 1895.

cards held between apparatus and screen made no perceptible difference. A single sheet of tin foil is scarcely noticeable; only after several layers have been laid on top of each other is a shadow clearly visible on the screen. Thick blocks of wood are also transparent; fir planks from 2 cm. to 3 cm. thick are but very slightly opaque. A film of aluminium about 15 mm. thick weakens the effect very considerably, though it does not entirely destroy the fluorescence. Several centimeters of vulcanized India-rubber let the rays through. Glass plates of the same thickness behave in a different way, according as they contain lead (flint glass) or not; the former are much less transparent than the latter. If the hand is held between the discharge tube and the screen, the dark shadow of the bones is visible within the slightly dark shadow of the hand. Water, bisulphide of carbon, and various other liquids behave in this respect as if they were very transparent.

By the "transparency" of a body I denote the ratio of the brightness of a fluorescent screen held right behind the body in question to the brightness of the same screen under exactly the same conditions, but without the interposing body.

For brevity's sake I should like to use the expression "rays" and to distinguish these from other rays I will call them "X rays." I was not able to determine whether water was more transparent than air. Behind plates of copper, silver, lead, gold, platinum, fluorescence is still clearly visible, but only when the plates are not too thick. Platinum 0.2 mm. thick is transparent; silver and copper sheets may be decidedly thicker. Lead 1.5 mm. thick is as good as opaque, and was on this account often made use of. A wooden rod of 20 by 20 mm. cross-section, painted white, with lead paint on one side, behaves in a peculiar manner. When it is interposed between apparatus and screen it has almost no effect when the X rays go through the rod parallel to the painted side, but it throws a dark shadow if the rays have to traverse the paint. Very similar to the metals themselves are their salts, whether solid or in solution.

(3) These experimental results and others lead to the conclusion that the transparency of different substances of the same thickness is mainly conditioned by their density; no other property is in the least comparable with this.

The following experiments, however, show that density is not altogether alone on its influence. I experimented on the transparency of nearly the same thickness of glass, aluminium, calcspar, and quartz. The density of these substances is nearly the same, and yet it was quite evident that the spar was decidedly less transparent than the other bodies, which were very much like each other in their behavior. I have not observed calcspar fluoresce in a manner comparable with glass.

(4) With increasing thickness all bodies become less transparent. In order to find a law connecting transparency with thickness, I made some photographic observations, the photographic plate being partly covered with an increasing number of sheets of tin foil. Photometric measurements will be undertaken when I am in possession of a suitable photometer.

(5) Sheets of platinum, lead, zinc, and aluminium were rolled until they appeared to be of almost equal transparency. The following table gives the thickness in millimeters, the thicknesses relative to the platinum and the density:

	Thickness.	Relative Thickness.	Density.
Pt.	0.018	1	21.5
Pb.	0.05	3	11.3
Zn.	0.10	6	7.1
Al.	3.5	200	2.6

It is to be observed, in connection with these figures, that although the product of the thickness into the density may be the same, it does not in any way follow that the transparency of the different metals is the same. The transparency increases at a greater rate than this product decreases.

(6) The fluorescence of barium-platino-cyanide is not the only recognizable phenomenon due to X rays. It may be observed, first of all, that other bodies fluoresce—for example, phosphorus, calcium compounds, uranium glass, ordinary glass, calcspar, rock salt, etc.

Of especial interest in many ways is the fact that photographic dry plates show themselves susceptible to X rays. We are thus in a position to corroborate many phenomena in which mistakes are easy, and I have, whenever possible, controlled each important ocular observation on fluorescence by means of photography. Owing to the property possessed by the rays passing almost without any absorption through thin sheets of wood, paper, or tin foil, we can take the impressions on the photographic plate inside the camera or paper cover while in a well-lit room. In former days this property of the ray only showed itself in the necessity under which we lay of not keeping undeveloped plates, wrapped in the usual .paper and board, for any length of time, in the vicinity of discharge tubes. It is still open to question whether the chemical effect on the silver salts of photographic plates is exercised directly by the X rays. It is possible that this effect is due to the fluorescent light which, as mentioned above, may be generated on the glass plate, or perhaps on the layer of gelatine. "Films" may be used just as well as glass plates.

I have not as yet experimentally proved that the X rays are able to cause thermal effects, but we may very well take their existence as probable, since it is proved that the fluorescent phenomenon alters the properties of X rays, and it is certain that all the incident X rays do not leave the bodies as such.

The retina of the eye is not susceptible to these rays. An eye brought close up to the discharge apparatus perceives nothing, although, according to experiments made, the media contained in the eye are fairly transparent.

(7) As soon as I had determined the transparency of different substances of various thicknesses, I hastened to ascertain how the X rays behaved when passed through a prism—whether they were refracted or not. Water and carbon disulphide, in prisms of about 30 degrees refractive angle, showed, neither with the fluorescing screen nor with the photographic plate, any sign of refraction. For purposes of comparison the refraction of light rays was observed under the same conditions; the refracted images on the plate were respectively about 10 mm. and 20 mm. from the non-refracted one. With an aluminium and a vulcanized rubber prism of 30 degrees angle I have obtained images on photographic plates in which one may perhaps see refraction. But the matter is very uncertain, and even if refraction exists, it is so small that the refractive index of the X ray for the above materials can only be, at the highest, 1.05. Using the fluorescent screen, I was unable to discover any refraction at all in the case of the aluminium and the rubber prism.

Researches with prisms of denser metals have yielded up to now no certain results, on account of the small transparency and consequently lessened intensity of the transmitted ray.

In view of this state of things, and the importance of the question whether X rays are refracted on passing from one medium to another, it is very satisfactory that this question can be attacked in another way than by means of prisms. Finely powdered substances in sufficient thicknesses only allow a very little of the incident light to pass through, and that is dispersed by the refraction and reflection. Now, powdered substances are quite as transparent to X rays as are solid bodies of equal mass. Hence it is proved that refraction and regular reflection do not exist to a noticeable degree. The experiments were carried out with finely-powdered rock salt, with pulverulent electrolytic silver, and with the zinc powder much used in chemical work. In no case was any difference observed between the transparency of the powdered and solid substance, either when using the fluorescent screen or the photographic plate.

It follows from what has been said that the X rays cannot be concentrated by lenses; a large vulcanized rubber and glass lens were without influence. The shadow of a round rod is darker in the middle than at the edge; that of a tube filled with any substance more transparent than the material of the tube is lighter in the middle than at the edge

(8) The question of the reflection of the X rays is settled in one's mind by the preceding paragraphs, and no appreciable regular reflection of the rays from the substances experimented with need be looked for. Other investigations, which I will describe here, lead to the same result. Nevertheless, an observation must be mentioned which at first sight appears to contradict the above statement. I exposed a photographic plate to the X rays, protected against light rays by black paper, the glass side being directed toward the discharge tube. The sensitive layer was nearly covered, star fashion, with blanks of platinum, lead, zinc and aluminium. On developing the negative it was clearly noticeable that the blackening under the platinum, lead, and especially under the zinc, was greater than in other places. The aluminium had exercised hardly any effect. It appeared, therefore, that the three above-mentioned metals had reflected the rays. Never-

theless other causes for the greater blackening were thinkable, and in order to make sure I made a second experiment, and laid a piece of thin aluminium, which is opaque to ultra-violet rays though very transparent to X rays, between the sensitive layers and the metal blanks. As again much the same result was found, a reflection of X rays by the above-mentioned metals was demonstrated. But if we connect these facts with the observation that powders are quite as transparent as solid bodies, and that, moreover, bodies with rough surfaces are, in regard to the transmission of X rays, as well as in the experiment just described, the same as polished bodies, one comes to the conclusion that regular reflection, as already stated, does not exist, but that the bodies behaved to the X rays as muddy media do to light.

Again, as I could discover no refraction at the point of passage from one medium to another, it would seem as if the X rays went through all substances at the same speed, and that in a medium which is everywhere, and in which the material particles are imbedded; the particles obstructing the propagation of the X rays in proportion to the density of the bodies.

(9) Hence it may be that the arrangement of the particles in the bodies influences the transparency; that, for example, equal thicknesses of calcspar would exhibit different transparencies according as the rays were in the direction of the axis or at right angles to it. Researches with calcspar and quartz have yielded a negative result.

(10) It is well known that Lenard, in his beautiful investigation on Hittorf cathode rays passed through thin aluminium foil, came to the conclusions that these rays were actions in the ether, and that they pass about my rays.

In his last work Lenard has determined the absorption co-efficient of various bodies for cathode rays; and among other things for air atmospheric pressure at 4.1, 3.4, 3.1, per centimeter, and found it connected with the exhaustion of the gas contained in the discharge apparatus. In order to estimate the discharge pressure by the spark-gap method, I used in my researches almost always the same exhaustion. I succeeded with a Weber photometer (I do not possess a better one) in comparing the intensity of the light of my fluorescing screen at distances of about 100 mm. and 200 mm. from the discharge apparatus, and found in the case of three tests agreeing well with one another that it varied very nearly inversely at the square of the distance of the screen from the discharge apparatus. Hence the air absorbs a very much smaller fraction of the X rays than of the cathode rays. This result is also quite in agreement with the result previously mentioned that the fluorescing light was still observable at a distance of two meters from the discharge apparatus.

Other bodies behave generally like air—that is to say, they are more transparent for X rays than for cathode rays.

(11) A further noteworthy difference in the behavior of cathode rays and X rays consists in the fact that, in spite of many attempts, I have not succeeded, even with very strong magnetic fields, in deflecting X rays by a magnet. The magnetic deflection has been up to now a characteristic mark of the cathode ray; it was, indeed, noticed by Hertz and Lenard that there were different kinds of cathode rays "distinguishable from one another by their phosphorescing powers, absorption and magnetic deflection," but a considerable deflection was nevertheless observed in all cases, and I do not think this characteristic will be given up without overwhelming evidence.

(12) After experiments bearing specially on this question it is certain that the spot on the wall of the discharge apparatus which fluoresces most decidedly must be regarded

as the principal point of the radiation of the X rays in all directions. The X rays thus start from the point at which, according to the researches of different investigators, the cathode rays impinge upon the wall of the glass tube. If one deflects the cathode rays within the apparatus by a magnet, it is found that the X rays are emitted from another spot—that is to say, from the new termination of the cathode stream.

On this account, also, the X rays, which are not deflected, cannot merely be unaltered reflected cathode rays passing through the glass wall. The greater density of the glass outside the discharge tube cannot, according to Lenard, be made responsible for the great difference in the "deflectability."

I therefore come to the conclusion that the X rays are not identical with the cathode rays, but that they are generated by the cathode rays at the glass wall of the discharge apparatus.

(13) This excitation does not only take place in glass, but also in aluminium, as I was able to ascertain with an apparatus closed by a sheet of aluminium 2 mm. thick. Other substances will be studied later on.

(14) The justification for giving the names of "rays" to the influence emanating from the wall of the discharge apparatus depends partly on the very regular shadows which they form when one interposes more or less transparent bodies between the apparatus and fluorescing screen or photographic plate. Many such shadow pictures, the formation of which possesses a special charm, have I observed—some photographically. For example, I possess photographs of the shadow of the profile of the door separating the room in which was the discharge apparatus from the room in which was the photographic plates; also photographs of the shadows of the bones of the hand, of the shadow of a wire wound on a wooden spool, of a weight

inclosed in a small box, of a compass in which the magnetic needle is completely surrounded by metal, of a piece of metal the lack of homogeneity of which was brought out by the X rays, etc.

To show the rectilinear propagation of the X rays there is a pin-hole photograph, which I was able to take by means of the discharge apparatus covered with black paper. The image is weak but unmistakably correct.

(15) I looked very carefully for interference phenomena with X rays, but unfortunately, perhaps only on account of the small intensity of the rays, without success.

(16) Researches to determine whether electrostatic forces affect X rays in any way have been begun, but are not completed.

(17) If we ask what X rays, which certainly cannot be cathode rays, really are, we are led at first sight, owing to their powerful fluorescing and chemical properties, to think of ultra-violet light. But we immediately encounter serious objections. If X rays be in reality ultra-violet light this light must possess the following characteristics:

(*a*) It must show no perceptible refraction on passing from air into water, bisulphide of carbon, aluminium, rock salt, glass, zinc, etc.

(*b*) It must not be regularly reflected to any appreciable extent from the above bodies.

(*c*) It must not be polarizable by the usual means.

(*d*) Its absorption must not be influenced by any of the properties of substances to the same extent as it is by their density.

In other words, we must assume that these ultra-violet rays behave in quite a different manner to any infra-red, visible, or ultro-violet rays hitherto known. I could not bring myself to this conclusion, and I have, therefore, sought another explanation.

There seems at least some connection between the new

rays and light rays in the shadow pictures and in the fluorescing and chemical activity of both kinds of rays. Now, it has been long known that besides the tranverse light vibrations, longitudinal vibrations might take place in the ether, and according to the view of different physicists must take place. Certainly their existence has not up till now been made evident, and their properties have not on that account been experimentally investigated.

May not the new rays be due to longitudinal vibrations in the ether?

I must admit that I have put more and more faith in this idea in the course of my research, and it behooves me, therefore, to announce my suspicion, although I know well that this explanation requires further corroboration.

As my investigations will have to be interrupted for several weeks, I propose, in the following paper, to communicate a few new results.[32]

(18) At the time of my first communication it was known to me that the X rays were able to discharge electrified bodies, and I suspected that it was X rays, not the unaltered cathode rays, which got through his aluminium window, that Lenard had to do with in connection with distant electrified bodies. When I published my researches, however, I decided to wait until I could communicate unexceptionable results. Such are only obtainable when one makes the observation in a space which is not only completely protected against the electrostatic influences of the vacuum tube, leading-in wires, induction coil, etc., but which is also protected against the air coming from the vicinity of the discharge apparatus. To this end I made a box of soldered sheet zinc large enough to receive me and the necessary apparatus, and which, even to an opening which could be closed by a zinc door, was quite

32 Second communication to Wurzburg Physico-Medical Society; Scientific American, May 30, 1896.

air-tight. The wall opposite the door was almost covered with lead. Near one of the discharge apparatus placed outside, the lead-covered zinc wall was provided with a slot 4 cm. wide, and the opening was then hermetically closed with a thin aluminium sheet. Through this window the X rays could come into the observation box. I have observed the following phenomena:

(*a*) Positively or negatively electrified bodies in air are discharged when placed in the path of X rays, and the more quickly the more powerful the rays. The intensity of the rays was estimated by their effect on a fluorescent screen or on a photographic plate. It is all the same whether the electrified bodies are conductors or insulators. Up to the present I have discovered no specific difference in the behavior of different bodies with regard to the rate of discharge, and the same remark applies to the behavior of positive and negative electricity. Nevertheless, it is not impossible that small differences exist.

(*b*) If an electric conductor is surrounded by a solid insulator, such as paraffine, instead of by air, the radiation acts as if the insulating envelope were swept by a flame connected to earth.

(*c*) If this insulating envelope is closely surrounded by a conductor connected to earth, which should like the insulator be transparent to X rays, the radiation, with the means at my disposal, apparently no longer acts on the inner electrified conductor.

(*d*) The observations described in *a*, *b*, and *c* tend to show that air traversed by X rays possesses the property of discharging electrified bodies with which it comes in contact.

(*e*) If this be really the case, and if, further, the air retains this property for some time after the X rays have been extinguished, it must be possible to discharge electrified bodies by such air, although the bodies themselves are not in the path of the rays.

It is possible to convince oneself in various ways that this actually happens. I will describe one arrangement, perhaps not the simplest possible. I employed a brass tube 3 cm. in diameter and 45 cm. long. A few centimeters from one end a portion of the tube was cut away and replaced by a thin sheet of aluminium. At the other end an insulated brass ball fastened to a metal rod was led into the tube through an air-tight gland. Between the ball and the closed end of the tube a side tube was soldered on, which could be placed in communication with an aspirator. When the aspirator was worked the brass ball was surrounded by air, which on its way through the tube went past the aluminium window. The distance from the window to the ball was over 20 cm. I arranged the tube in the zinc box in such a manner that the X rays passed through the aluminium window at right angles to the axis of the tube, so that the insulated ball was beyond the reach of the rays in the shadow. The tube and the zinc box were connected together; the ball was connected to a Hankel electroscope. It was seen that a charge (positive or negative) communicated to the ball was not affected by the X rays so long as the air in the tube was at rest, but the charge immediately diminished considerably when the aspirator caused the air traversed by the rays to stream past the ball. If the ball by being connected to accumulators was kept at a constant potential, and if air which had been traversed by the rays was sucked through the tube, an electric current was started as if the ball had been connected with the wall of the tube by a bad conductor.

(*f*) It may be asked in what way the air loses this property communicated to it by the rays. Whether it loses it as time goes on, without coming into contact with other bodies, is still doubtful. It is quite certain, on the other hand, that a short disturbance of the air by a body of large surface, which need not be electrified, can render the air inoperative. If one pushes, for example, a sufficiently thick plug of cotton wool so far into the tube that the air which has been traversed by the rays must stream through the cotton wool before it reaches the ball, the charge of the ball remains unchanged when suction is commenced. If the plug is placed right in front of the aluminium window the result is the same as if there were no cotton wool, a proof that dust particles are not the cause of the observed discharge. Wire gauze acts in the same way as cotton wool, but the meshes must be very small and several layers must be placed one over the other if we want the air to be active. If the nets are not connected to earth, as heretofore, but connected to a constant potential source of electricity, I have always observed what I expected; however, these investigations are not concluded.

(*g*) If the electrified bodies are placed in dry hydrogen instead of air they are equally discharged. The discharge in hydrogen seems to me somewhat the slower. This observation is not, however, very reliable, on account of the difficulty of securing equally powerful X rays in successive experiments. The method of filling the apparatus with hydrogen precluded the possibility of the thin layer of air which clings to the surface of the bodies at the commencement playing an appreciable part in connection with the discharge.

(*h*) In highly-exhausted vessels the discharge of a body in the path of the X rays takes place far slower —in one case it was, for instance, 70 times slower—than in the same vessels when filled with air or hydrogen at atmospheric pressure.

(*i*) Experiments on the behavior of a mixture of chlorine and hydrogen, when under the influence of the X rays, have been commenced.

(*j*) Finally, I should like to mention that the results of

the investigations on the discharging property of the X rays, in which the influence of the surrounding gases was not taken into account, should be for the most part accepted with reserve.

(19) In many cases it is of advantage to put in circuit between the X ray producer and the Ruhmkorff coil a Tesla condenser and transformer. This arrangement has the following advantages: Firstly, the discharge apparatus gets less hot, and there is less probability of its being pierced; secondly, the vacuum lasts longer, at least this was the case with my apparatus; and thirdly, the apparatus produces stronger X rays. In apparatus which was either not sufficiently or too highly exhausted to allow the Ruhmkorff coil alone to work well, the use of a Tesla transformer was of great advantage.

The question now arises—and I may be permitted to mention it here, though I am at present not in a position to give an answer to it—whether it is possible to generate X rays by means of a continuous discharge at a constant discharge potential, or whether oscillations of the potential are invariably necessary for their production.

(20) In paragraph 13 of my first communication it was stated that X rays not only originate in glass but also in aluminium. Continuing my researches in this direction, I have found no solid bodies incapable of generating X rays under the influence of cathode rays. I know of no reason why liquids and gases should not behave in the same way.

Quantitative differences in the behavior of different bodies have, however, revealed themselves. If, for example, we let the cathode rays fall on a plate, one half consisting of a 0.3 mm. sheet of platinum and the other half of a 1 mm. sheet of aluminium, a pin-hole photograph of this double plate will show that the sheet of platinum emits a far greater number of X rays than does the aluminium sheet, this remark applying in either case to the side upon which the cathode rays impinge. From the reverse side of the platinum, however, practically no X rays are emitted, but from the reverse side of the aluminium a relatively large number are radiated. It is easy to construct an explanation of this observation, still it is to be recommended that before so doing we should learn a little more about the characteristics of X rays.

It must be mentioned, however, that this fact has a practical bearing. Judging by my experience up to now, platinum is the best for generating the most powerful X rays. I used a few weeks ago, with excellent results, a discharge apparatus in which a concave mirror of aluminium acted as cathode and a sheet of platinum as anode, the platinum being at an angle of 45 degrees to the axis of the mirror and at the center of curvature.

(21) The X rays in this apparatus start from the anode. I conclude from experiments with variously-shaped apparatus that as regards the intensity of the X rays it is a matter of indifference whether or not the spot at which these rays are generated be the anode. With special attention to researches with alternate currents from a Tesla transformer, a discharge apparatus is being made in which both electrodes are concave aluminium mirrors, their axes being at right angles; at the common center of curvature there is a "cathode-ray catching" sheet of platinum. As to the utility of this apparatus I will report further at a later date.

CHAPTER III.

PROFESSOR ROENTGEN, in his report, Section 1, Chapter II., refers to an apparatus used in his discovery of the X rays, and giving currents of very high potential, necessary to charge a Crookes' or vacuum tube, called an induction or Rhumkorff coil.

We have been familiarized with the properties of magneto-induction of Volta and Ampère, the phenomenon of which was, that when the pole of a magnet was presented to a closed solenoid of insulated wire a momentary current was established in the coil, and that by withdrawing the magnet another momentary current in the opposite direction was occasioned.

This law is the fundamental principle of our modern electrical technic.

Later came the discovery of Faraday (Chapter I., Part II.), the discovery of the induced current, and still later the property of increased potential in the induced or secondary current, as being enormously multiplied to that of the initial or primary circuit.

The value of induction has been fully described in dealing with electro-dynamics, in the discoveries of Pixii, Clarke, Page, and Stöhrer, wherein the rapid rotation of an armature containing coils of insulated wire, before the faces or poles of the maguet, created currents of considerable potential.

The induction coil, however, although of the same class, differs from this so-called class of frictional electrical magneto-induction machine, in that its induced currents depend upon contact rapidly made and broken, as mentioned on page heretofore in refering to the vibrator or rheotome.

The first practical spark induction coil was made by Professor Rhumkorff. It was about 24 inches long. The largest induction coil made, was that of Spottiswoode, in 1876.[33] The weight of the apparatus was 750 kilograms; the length of the containing cylinders 120 centimeters, and the outer diameter of the same 50 centimeters. The inner spool containing the core weighed 25 kilograms; the copper wire used had a diameter of 2½ millimeters and was 604 meters long, wound in 1,334 turns, in 6 layers.

The outer spool contained 240 miles, or 426 kilometers, of wire. The windings were made in four sections, the first two containing wire of a diameter of ¼ millimeter, while the other two were somewhat heavier. The entire number of turns in the secondary were 341,850. The sparking distance of this apparatus depended upon the primary circuit employed. The following gives his results:

A battery of 5 groove cells gave a spark of 71 centimeters; 10 groove cells, 88 centimeters; 30 groove cells, 107 centimeters.

However, we will describe the ordinary Rhumkorff induction apparatus most suitable for X ray work.

The primary coil is built on the principle of the electromagnet. The core or magnet, well insulated, contains the windings of rather heavy cotton-covered wire—No. 12 B. W. G. It is composed of soft iron wires, No. 30 B. W. G. —used preferably to the solid bar, for the reason that it intensifies the primary current and permits rapid magnetization and demagnetization. The proportion of the core length to the sparking distance of the secondary coil is about as follows: ½-inch spark discharge, $4\frac{3}{4} \times \frac{10}{16}$ inch core

33 From description in "Philosophical Magazine," London, January, 1877; Wildermann, Grundl. der Elek., p. 94.

dimensions; 1-inch spark discharge, $8 \times \frac{3}{4}$ inch core dimensions; 2-inch spark discharge, $9 \times \frac{11}{16}$ inch core dimensions; 6-inch spark discharge, $19 \times 1\frac{1}{2}$ inches core dimensions.

Heavy copper wire is preferred for the primary coil on account of its low resistance.

The primary voltage is very small and the amperage considerably greater—from 4 to 12 amperes. It is therefore

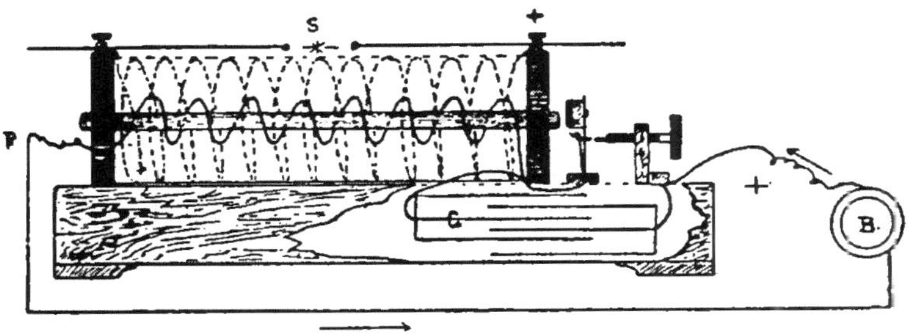

FIG. 29.

necessary to have as little resistance as possible—a few turns of wire would be sufficient. (Fig. 29.)

The crude file rheotome mentioned before is replaced by the Wagnerian hammer or automatic circuit breaker, for the purpose of causing rapid interruptions in the primary circuit. It is composed of a flat German silver spring having at its upper and inner end a piece of iron somewhat larger than the diameter of the core, fastened to it, termed its "head" and placed directly in front of the primary core, with enough space between the two to allow of free vibration. The lower end of the spring is fastened to the case upon which the entire apparatus is mounted.

Just above the center, and to its outer side, a rivet of platinum is inserted, against which the screw adjustment, containing another piece of platinum, rests.

Platinum is used to prevent, as far as is possible, the sparking caused by the heavy currents jumping across at these points when the spring vibrates.

It is very essential, in order to obtain the best induction, to obtain a clean, rapid make-and-break. The sparking, however, would use up considerable current in producing heat and light, so that it has been found necessary to use a condenser.

The condensers usually used are made of alternate layers of 50 to 200 sheets of tin foil, 8x8 inches, separated by clean paraffined paper, of from 4 to .007th of an inch in thickness and about an inch larger than the sheets of foil laid between each pair of sheets. The corners of the foil are alternately joined in multiple, and each collective set connected to the circuit breaker, as shown in Fig. 29. Care must be taken that no connections exist between the two sets of tin foil, as that would short circuit the rheotome and no effect would be obtained in the coil.

The condenser temporarily stores the electrical energy—the amount stored depending upon its capacity, measured by the micro-farad; a .000001th part of the capacity of a body raised to the potential of one volt by a charge of one ampere, for one second, at one volt, which would equal one coloumb.

The original form of the condenser, as we know, was the leyden jar already described. The condenser stores the current when made or broken, but unloads faster than it loads up, owing to the heavy current flowing when the circuit is broken, occasioned by the inductive influence of one turn of wire upon its neighboring turn.

The head of the hammer opposite the end of the core works toward and away from the latter in vibrating—the circuit coming from the battery through the screw to the spring, from the spring to the primary coil, and then back to the battery. This constitutes the complete primary current.

The passage of the current through the primary coil magnetizes the core, which attracts the hammer, drawing the spring away from the platinum contact in the screw, and so on, over and over again.

This simple form of contact breaker, automatic circuit breaker, vibrator or rheotome, however, has its disadvantages as its vibrations are limited to a certain rate and not suitable for heavy currents. Such as they are, their rate of vibration differs even when low currents are used.

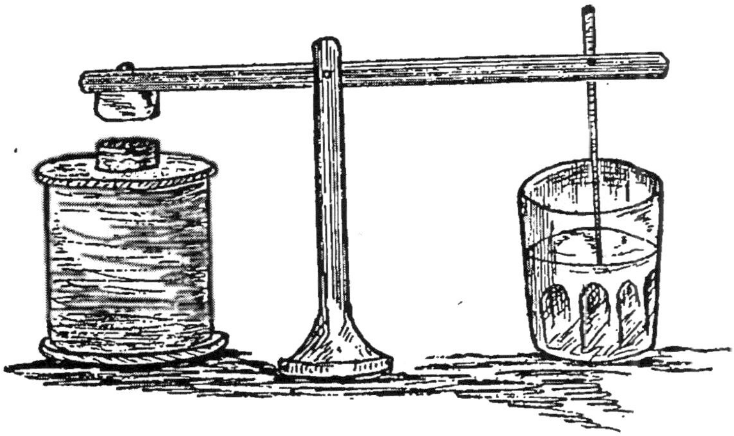

Fig. 30.

And again a decisive make-and-break is all-important in the production of X rays, and the main defect in this class of rheotomes is their tendency to vibrate sinusoidally, causing irregularity and a weakened effect.

When in action all circuit breakers give out a musical note of definite tone. Faraday observed that the tone would indicate the number of the vibrations of the spring.

For the value of notes and the number of vibrations necessary to produce them, the author refers the reader to a standard work on acoustics. The form of vibrator usually used on the very large coils is of the mercury type.[34] (Fig. 30.)

A metal upright holds a pivoted arm with an armature,

34 See description in "Practical Radiography," Snowden Ward, London.

which is attracted by the core of a magnetic coil. Below and on the other end of the arm is placed a platinum point or needle, adjustable by a set-screw, to the desired length. The needle dips down into a glass cup containing a quantity of metallic mercury, floated with a layer of spirits of turpentine. The latter, being a non-conductor, outs out the sparking which would naturally occur at this place as the needle is raised, not unlike the sparking of the rheotomes already described.

The current from the battery flows to the mercury in the cup, through the needle, along the arm, down the upright, through the primary coil, and back to the battery. As the current excites the magnet it draws the armature to it and raises the needle out of the mercury, so breaking the current and demagnetizing the core, releasing the armature by the aid of a spring, again allowing the needle to dip into the mercury, making contact, etc.

But even this rheotome, although accurate, does not give the necessary number of interruptions. For that reason, another form has been invented in the form of the make-and-break wheel.[35] The latter consists of a round disk or wheel of brass, about 6 inches in diameter and ½ inch thick, having a number of pieces of slate or fiber mounted in its periphery. A brush is placed in contact with the outer rim, to collect the current from the metal spaces, as the disk is made to revolve.

A second brush is placed in contact with the outer border of a second and smaller wheel, permanently fixed to the side of the former, which is made of brass only, allowing the current to flow through it from the brush, and having no insulated pieces set into its periphery, permits of a constant and even conduction of the primary current to its larger fellow.

---

35 Pupin: Lect. N. Y. Acad. Sci., April 6, 1896; "Science," New York, April 10, 1896.

As the wheel rotates, the current is made as the upper brush comes in contact with the metal of the wheel, and broken when passing over the slate. The entire wheel, or rather pair of wheels, is mounted upon the shaft of an ordinary electric motor of about one horse power. The surface of the large wheel should be kept carefully polished, to prevent the brushes from carrying the metal of the wheel proper over the slate, so preventing a break of the current.

As many as 50,000 makes-and-breaks per minute can be obtained in this way. (Fig. 31.)

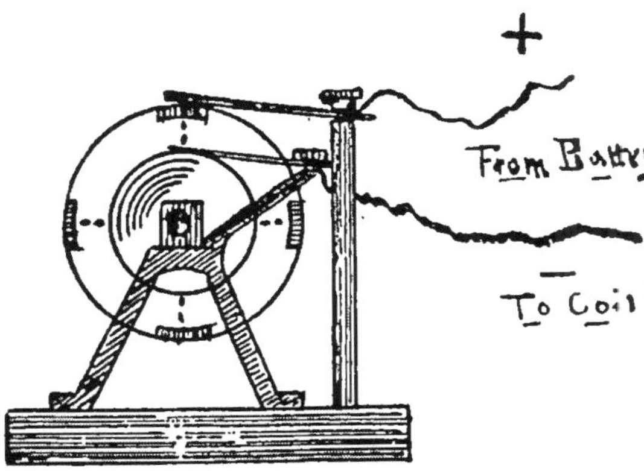

FIG. 31.

Condensers are used as in the usual way, and it has been found that an increase of their capacity or micro-farads tends to cut out or reduce sparking at the brushes to a minimum. From 2 to 25 micro-farads can be employed, according to the dimensions and spark discharge of the coil.

The sectional condensers of Marshall are exceedingly useful, as their capacity can be reduced or increased at will. As the primary currents can be made very heavy, it may be necessary to mount an air blast or Root blower with insulated tongue in connection with the rotary rheotome. The tongue of the former is placed directly over the point of contact of the upper brush, to blow or cut out the sparking which would naturally occur here.

The air blast can be run by the same motor, or another motor can be used, connected to it by a belt.

The author recommends this form of rheotome to those who have the advantage of having a public current in their offices or laboratories, as the results are far better than those obtained with the ordinary rheotome.

To see the human heart beat would certainly require such an affair, although the mercury interrupter may suffice where an exceedingly good tube and screen is used.

So much then for the primary current.

The secondary circuit is very simple. It has been found that by considerably multiplying the turns of wire—which in this case are very fine indeed and most carefully insulated—in proportion to the primary coil, the greater will the potential and the smaller the amperage of the secondary coil be. As the X rays require a current of very high voltage, a great deal of wire is necessary, and thousands of feet constitute the windings—the amount depending upon the size of the coil. About 1¼ pounds of No. 36 B. W. G. are necessary for each inch of spark.

One can readily imagine the current necessary to overcome the resistance of the atmosphere and give sparks from 1 to 12 inches in length.

For a comparison of the primary and secondary coils refer to the dimension of the Spottiswoode coil.

The secondary coil has its terminals soldered to binding posts, positive and negative, usually found mounted on top of the reel ends. These should be high and clearing the outside of the coil considerably, to prevent sparking from the pole to the core or primary coil.

The discharger is made to determine the distance of the spark discharge and consists of two sliding rods of brass, having at their outer ends insulated rubber handles and passing through the lower opening of the binding posts. The space between the dischargers, or that through which the spark travels, becomes the spark gap.

In turning on the primary current, a humming sound will be noticed, caused by the vibrator, and a crackling sparking discharge at the secondary poles will be noticed. By drawing the terminals or dischargers apart, the sparking distance increases in length and finally refuses to pass. By approximating the balls or points of the latter, we can determine exactly what length of spark discharge the coil will give.

The induced current of the secondary coil is found to be very powerful indeed, and it is advisable to keep all uninsulated material, as well as your hands, away from it, as dangerous results may follow heavy shocks. A 1¼-inch spark discharge should be the limit for physical treatment.

The current from the secondary coil, as you may expect, is alternating, but there is a greater impulse in one direction than in the other, which is due to the induced electromotive force in the secondary coil being much stronger at the break, and weaker at the make, of the primary current.

The cathode is usually spoken of as the preponderating pole, depending, however, upon the course of the primary circuit; therefore the sparks are discharged from that pole, the current being too feeble at the make to return the sparks from the other or anode to the cathode. That is why the sparks travel in but one direction.

In working with a spark coil it is not advisable to leave the dischargers beyond their sparking distance, as it causes considerable strain on the secondary insulation.

The tubes are connected to the secondary terminals, as will be described in the chapter on practical radiography.

The peculiar odor noticed when working with the discharge or spark coil in the air is due to ozone (O_3) or triatomic oxygen, brought about by a chemical action of the spark upon the atmosphere.

The sparks from the secondary terminals are not given off in straight lines, but assume a peculiar zigzag course, resembling lightning flashes. This is probably caused by the floating particles in the atmosphere, which have a tendency to draw or conduct the spark away from its course. In very low vacua the spark travels in straight lines.

The short, fat spark is called the calorific or heat spark. It is of a yellowish-red color, possibly due to the combustion of sodium in the atmosphere.

The spark discharge between balls is much noisier than when crossing between points of the secondary terminals, a fact described by Professor Niaudet,[36] of France.

The voltage of the secondary current, according to Gordon and Alexander Siemens, reckoned by the length of spark in air, is 33,000 volts per cubic centimeters between ball dischargers. If the discharge occurs between points, a greater length is obtained, with lower voltage, however, —reckoned at from 20 to 25,000 volts per centimeter of spark discharge. A 6-inch spark between two discharging secondary terminals would indicate about 300,000 volts.

THE INFLUENCE OR STATIC MACHINE.

The static machine and its principle has been somewhat fully described in Chapter I., on frictional electricity. However, as the static machine has found some favor with a number of experimenters, it may be well to briefly describe its applicaion to radiography.[37]

Although there are a number of influence machines made, all are modifications, more or less, of the Tölpler-Holtz, Wimshurst, etc., machine.

The Wimshurst has a great advantage over any other

---

36 Wildermann's Grundl. der Elect., p. 97.

37 Prof. Pupin, "Electricity," New York, Feb. 19, 1896; Rice: "Tube Energized by Wimshurst Machine," Elect. Eng., New York, April 22, 1896.

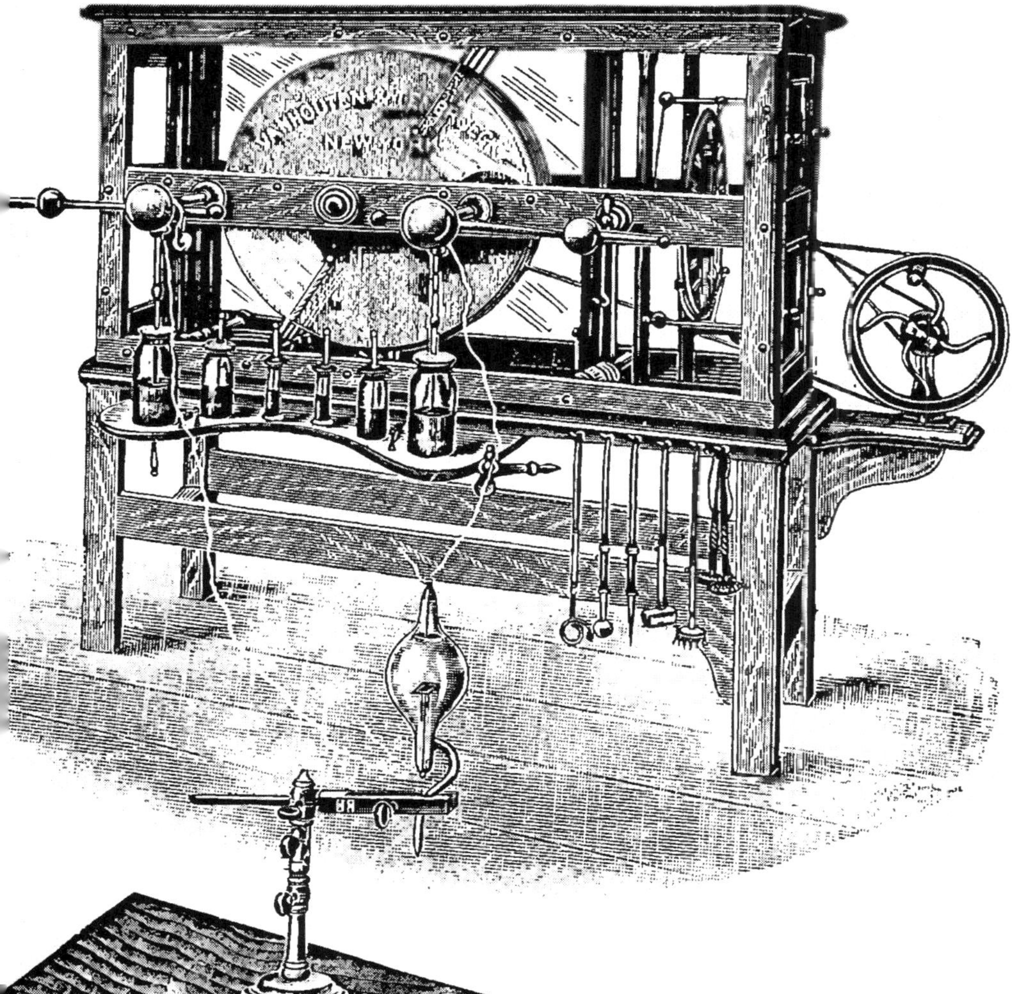

INFLUENCE, OR STATIC MACHINE OF THE LATEST TYPE, WITH EIGHT THIRTY-INCH REVOLVING PLATES RUNNING ON BALL BEARINGS AND HAVING THE WIMSHURST EXCITER ATTACHMENT. THE CONNECTIONS TO THE TUBE ARE HEREIN SHOWN.

apparatus in its economy. It is cheap, as compared to the complex Tölpler-Holtz apparatus, and from another point of view, no induction coil is needed. The Wimshurst machine has been successfully used by many, but there are precautions to observe, which must at all times be considered. Dr. Lawson Russell,[38] of England, gives the following rules:

(1) "Have the temperature of the experimenting room at not less than 65 degrees F., and the apparatus placed before a good fire or stove. The air of the room must be free from dust and moisture.

(2) "The Wimshurst, besides being warm, must, like air, be free from dust and adherent moisture. Its conducting rods should be in the position of greatest efficiency—that is, they should be at right angles with each other, and should form an angle of 45 degrees with fixed collectors. It should stand firmly and be driven steadily.

(3) "The wires between the machine and the tube should be fixed to the terminal electrodes or discharger close to the balls; they should be short, perfectly insulated, and the contact at the various connections should be perfect. If the wires are carried over or supported by anything in their way to the tube, let it be glass.

(4) "The typical tube for use with the Wimshurst is one of small dimensions, having a very high vacuum. It should be perfectly insulated, and on a steady stand. Heat the tube before the fire or with a spirit lamp, before beginning the exposure, and if, during the exposure, the current shows the slightest disinclination to pass through the tube, stop and heat the tube with a spirit lamp. If the tube be one having a very high vacuum, this may require to be done every half-minute. The make of tube best adapted for use with the Wimshurst is, I find, that known as the focus tube."

38 "Practical Radiography," Ward, London, p. 59.

No doubt if these directions are carried out to the letter the experimenter will obtain excellent results. Unfortunately moisture plays an important part in most all laboratories, caused not by damp cellars but by the sudden changes of our climate.

As to a fire in the laboratory, that is a rarity. Most laboratories are quite cool, especially those of experimenters, and the author will never forget the cold February and March nights, and the early morning hours of experimenting when warmth was little thought of.

A word about the connections of these machines. After determining the positive and negative poles, which you know are charged by induction, it is necessary to connect each pole—positive and negative—to a condenser, using a small pint size leyden jar. A discharge from larger jars has a tendency to crack the tube. The smaller jars give higher oscillations, estimated at about .000010ths per second, and although the size of the jar used is governed by the degree of vacuum in the tube, the given size usually answers the purpose very well.

The two coatings of tin foil are described as the internal armature (inner coating) and the external armature (outer coating). Connect the prime conductors to the internal armature and the external to wires to the vacuum tube.

Mr. E. W. Rice,[39] Technical Director of the General Electric Company, found that by omitting the jars the generation of current was practically non-intermittent, and advises the tube connection directly to the prime, or positive, and negative conductors of the static machine as in Fig. 32.

When the plate of the machine is turned by the aid of the handle, the current will pass from the prime conductor to the internal armature, so that the wire connected to

39 "The Wimshurst Machine," Elect. Eng., New York, April 22, 1896.

the external armature must be connected to the negative pole of the tube, and *vice versa* on the other side.

The length of the spark gap when using the small jars should be about 2 or 3 inches, unless the vacuum of the tube is sufficiently high to warrant a wider gap.

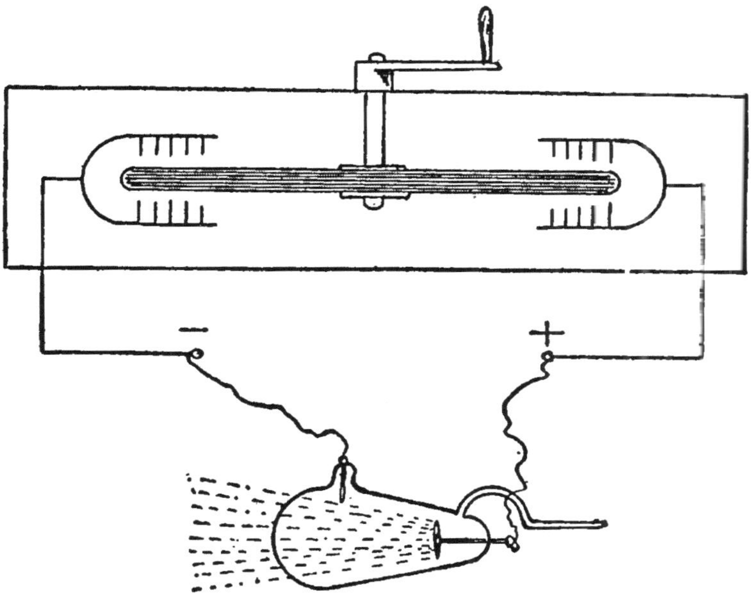

Fig. 32.

The experimenter will soon learn how to regulate the latter by experience. Dr. Morton [40] recommends that the spark gap be inclosed within an ebonite cylinder with closed ends, affording relief to the eye, ear and brain—as the sparkling and crackling sound is very annoying to the patient and can be obviated considerably by this method.

The power necessary to run such a machine is about $\frac{1}{8}$ to $\frac{1}{6}$ horse power. The most suitable source of power is the water or the electric motor.

40 "Photography of the Invisible," p. 83.

THE TESLA TRANSFORMER.

Professor Roentgen admits in his report (§ 19) the advantages obtained by employing a Tesla transformer within the secondary circuit of the Ruhmkorff coil. Mr. Tesla's experiments were certainly marvelous.

The X rays coming from tubes charged by his apparatus affected photographic plates at a distance of 60 feet. Although his apparatus is far too complicated to describe in so limited a space, we are nevertheless amply repaid by reading a short description of the modified apparatus which can be connected in circuit with any street alternating electric light current, by using a cut-down transformer giving 52 cr 104 volts. This is connected directly to the primary of the Tesla discharger, or, when used with the spark coil, the secondary terminals of the spark coil are connected to two condensers of very small size, highly insulated by immersion in oil.

Between the leads of the condenser is placed the spark gap, composed of two metallic balls; or, the Tesla discharger can be used and placed as near together as required for the effect desired. The condenser's secondary terminals are connected with the primary of the disruptive coil, composed of a glass or rubber tube, upon which about 60 turns of No. 18 gutta-percha-covered wire is wound. Note that the primary may be either inside or outside. In the illustration it is the outer coil, having four terminals—two going out to the condenser and two to the discharger.

The secondary coil fits into the former one in this case, and is composed of about 300 turns of No. 30 silk-covered magnetic wire wound upon a hard rubber or glass tube of about ½ inch in diameter. The terminals of this are connected to the vacuum tube. (Fig. 33.)

The entire disrupter or Tesla high-frequency transformer is immersed like the condensers in boiled-down linseed oil.

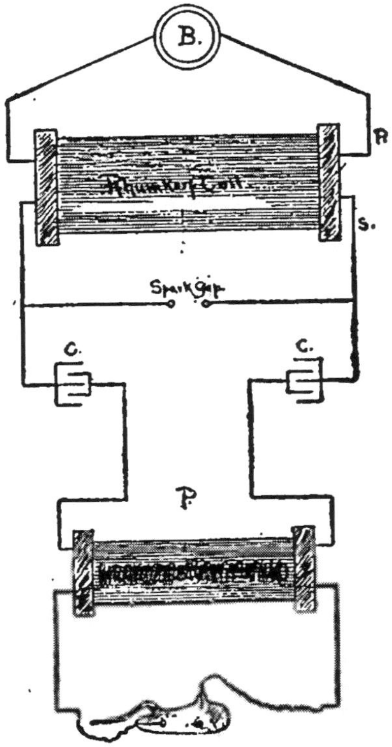

FIG. 33.

The circuit gives a very high luminosity to the vacuum tube. The oscillations of the current given by this apparatus are very rapid and of exceedingly high frequency of alternation.[41]

41 "Construction of High Frequency Coil of Tesla and Thomson;" see Description by Prof. A. F. McKissick, Am. Electrician, August, 1896; N. Y. Medical Journal, Sept. 5, 1897; "High Frequency Apparatus—Inventions of Tesla," etc., Martin.

CHAPTER IV.

THE VACUUM TUBE.[42]

FOR years, and ever since the time of Crookes' discovery of radiant matter, vacuum tubes of all descriptions have been made; all with but one purpose, and that to study the cathode ray. You have seen some of the modifications and the ingenious tube of Hertz and Lenard, likewise some of the original tubes devised by Crookes, illustrated in Chapter I., Part II.

But it would require many volumes, perhaps, to describe all. However, we will only consider the tubes necessary for X ray work, their construction, size and uses.

First, we have the ordinary Crookes' tube as used by Professor Roentgen in the discovery of the X rays, containing a very high vacuum—.000001th degree of atmospheric pressure, or one millionth part of the air as originally contained in the tube before being exhausted, equal to 0.00076 mm., 1315.789 millionths of an atmosphere equaling 1 mm.

These tubes are exhausted by combined hydraulic and mercury pumps. They have a small tube at one end, by which they are mounted on the pump receiver. When a sufficient vacuum is reached this is melted off by the aid of a Bunsen flame. A low vacuum tube would have the

42 See also "Radiant Matter," by William Crookes, in four parts, in Electrical Engineer, New York, Feb. 19 to March 11, 1896.

ordinary vacuum of 1,000, as contained in Geissler tubes, etc.

The glass used for most tubes is German soda-flint glass. This gives an apple-green color when subjected to the fluorescent properties of the X rays under vacuum. Other kinds of glass fluoresce in different colors.

The tube contains electrodes, so-called, to which the connections from the electric apparatus are made. These are of a number of shapes and sizes, but usually a tube contains two or three, one called the positive or anode and the other the negative or cathode.

The usual shape of these electrodes is either a rod or disk of platinum. Later aluminium has been employed in the form of concave mirrors, as described hereafter. The electrodes are fused into the glass walls of the tube, having a small ring at their outer end for connections. Platinum is preferable for fusing into the glass; when heated it expands at about the same rate as glass, avoiding cracking the latter.

The inner portion can be made of any metal, but platinum seems to be the favorite, although aluminium is used considerably, the only difficulty with the former being that when heated by the current it gives off a considerable amount of air, with a possibility of reducing the tube's vacuum, lessening the X ray emanations. The cooling of the metal would, however, take up some of the air given off.

The best form of aluminium to use is the electrolyzed. By this is meant a wire or disk that has been previously brought to a white heat by being subjected to a high electrical current, which drives off all of the superfluous air from its interstices. A peculiarity is that it becomes hardened by this process, as in fact most metals do.

Its advantage is, that when used within the tube it does not disintegrate as quickly as platinum. This is evidenced after the tube containing the platinum disks has been used for some time the glass becomes blackened from the deposit of the disintegrated metallic particles upon the walls of the tube.

Fig. 34 represents the familiar pear-shaped tube usually

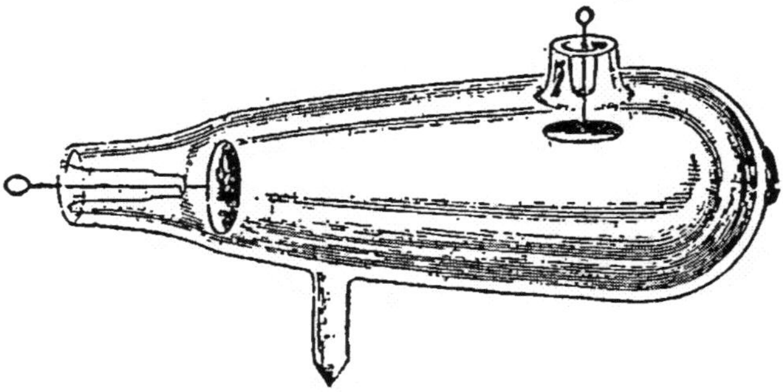

FIG. 34

used, having two disks or electrodes, one positive and the other negative. With this form of tube all of the early X ray work or results were accomplished, although many had tubes made after their own design. (Fig. 35.)

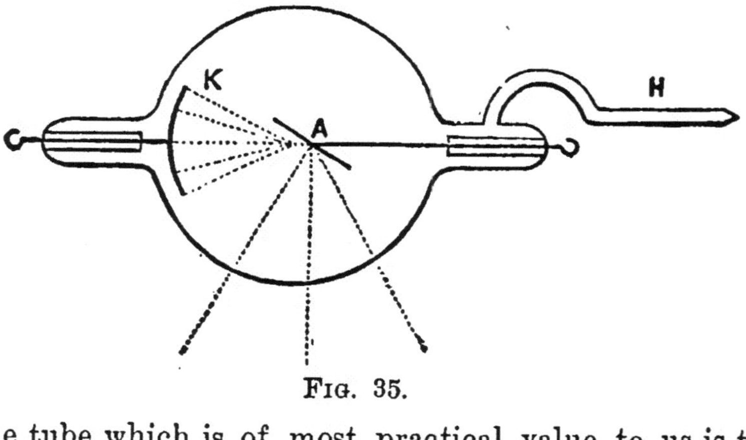

FIG. 35.

The tube which is of most practical value to us is the so-called focus tube, originally described and made by Shallenberger.[43] But its originality is also claimed by Herbert Jackson, of King's College,[44] London, and by Roentgen, himself, in his communication of March 7, 1896.

43 Elect. World, New York, March 7, 1896.

44 Elect. Review, London, March 13, 1896; Scientific American, April 4, 1896.

The cathode is made in the form of a concave mirror of aluminium, while the anode is a square disk of platinum, with its plane so placed as to act as a reflector, as it were, to the cathode rays produced, striking the plate at an angle of 45 degrees and throwing them outward to the glass and through the thin wall of the tube.

A similar tube, under the name of Newton focus tube, was imported from London by myself and received on the 20th day of March, through Muller & Co., New York. The author believes it to have been one of the first used in this country. The radiographs exhibited by me at the National Electrical Exposition, New York, May, 1896, were mostly made with this form of tube.

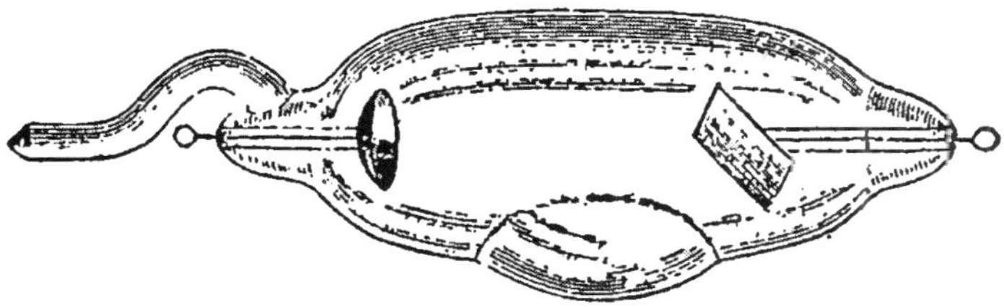

FIG. 36.

Fig. 36 shows a modification of the focus tube made after drawings by the author subjected to E. Greiner, of New York, and used by him with excellent results. It is somewhat larger than the former, allowing the use of higher potential currents, which have a tendency to jump across the outer surface of the tube, the danger of which is cracking of the tube. This has been remedied by making the external electrodes from 8 to 10 inches apart instead of $4\frac{1}{2}$ as in the Newton tube.

The tube is not blown so thin, but has a concavity extending outward, directly opposite the anode, and corresponding to a great extent to the peripheral area of the hemisphere of radiation. The concave portion is blown to a thickness of $\frac{1}{74}$ of an inch, and as the rays strike the glass at an angle is not liable to heat.

The following figure is that of a combined or double

focus tube originally described by Prof. Elihu Thomson,[45] and termed by him the "Standard." It is very suitable for high alternating or oscillating currents, and especially designed for the static machine, in which they are used as follows: The two outer ends or cathodes are connected to the prime conductor and the V-shaped platinum anode to the negative conductor.

When used with the spark coil the tube is quite economical, as only one cathode and anode are used. In the event of the breaking off of one of the outer rings—which often happens, as these tubes are necessarily delicate—the tube can be reversed and used at once. Another advantage is that when the vacuum becomes high from continual use the two outer cathode poles may be connected to the positive wire and charged, with the result of lowering the vacuum within a few moments. (Fig. 37.)

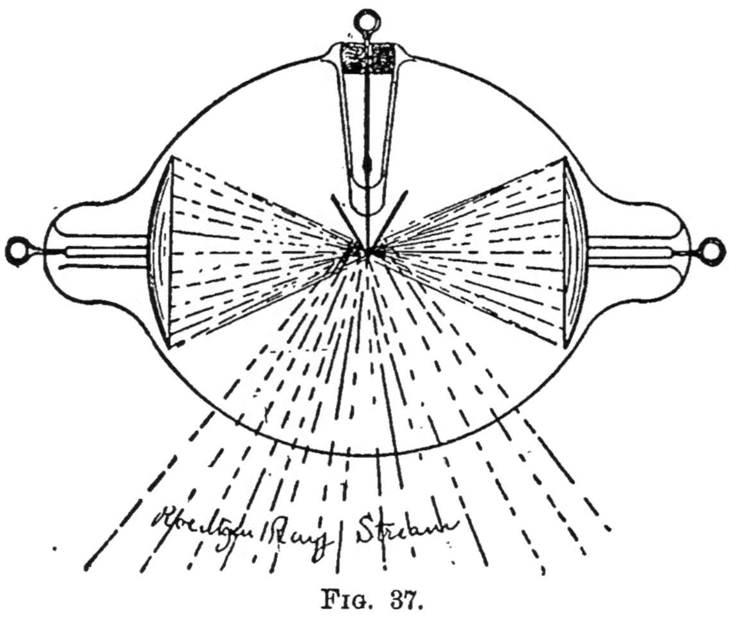

FIG. 37.

Tesla used a tube with but one electrode. They are especially devised for Tesla currents of exceedingly high frequency and potential.

45 Elect. Review, New York, April 15, 1896.

Edison devised a very ingenious tube, wherein the platinum plates or disks act as reflectors to one another. The form of the tube certainly promises exceedingly good results, and is especially adapted for use with the spark coil.

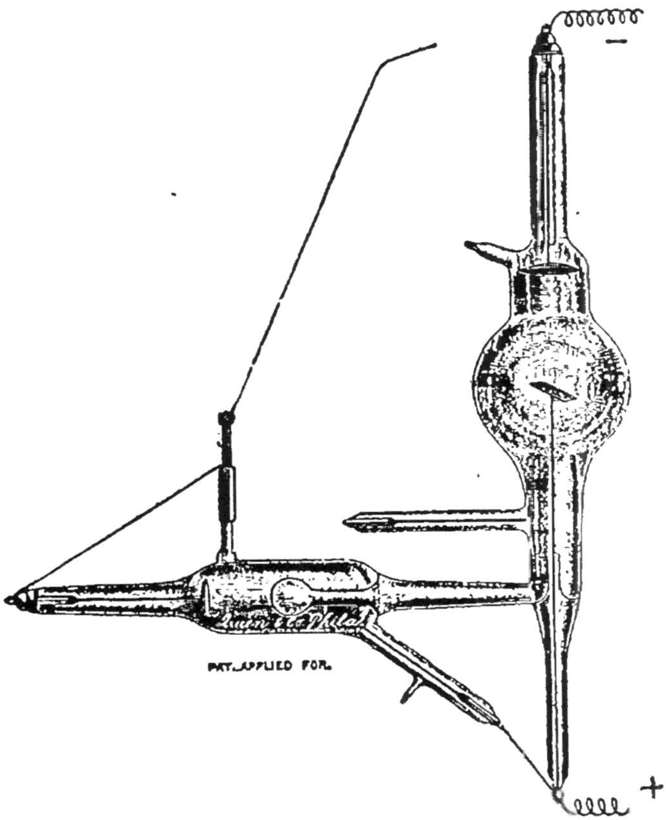

FIG. 38.

A great advance in the usefulness of tubes was made when the adjustable vacuum tube was perfected.

A number of these self-regulating tubes can be found in the market. The author has used the Queen tube in his hospital work lately and can recommend it as having distinct advantages over the non-adjustable tubes, the principal one having that of long life. (See Fig. 38.)

In the illustration a small bulb will be seen. This contains a metallic salt which gives off vapor when heated, re-absorbing it when cooling. It is a part of the main tube and surrounded by an auxiliary tube containing a low vacuum. The cathode electrode is placed opposite the small bulb, in such a way that when a current is passed through the low vacuum of the former, the latter is heated and its contained chemical is made to give out its confined vapor, so lessening the high vacuum of the large tube. The auxiliary tube is connected in shunt with the larger tube by its prolongated cathode. This becomes a brass wire without the tube, and is so made that it can be brought to or from the cathode pole of the main tube. It is only necessary to bring the shunt wire within sparking distance of the latter to cause a passage of sparks between the poles of the auxiliary tube. The proper vacuum can be obtained in a few seconds. The sparking across the shunt gap will cease, as the current passes through the larger tube. This actually makes the tube self-regulating, and guarantees a much longer life than the tube not provided with this arrangement.

Professor Pupin, during the early months following the discovery of Roentgen, used a tube without any electrodes within the tube, but substituted them with a piece of tin foil for the anode and cathode, fixed externally to the tube wall by rubber bands. The plaques of foil were connected to the terminals of the coil. With this kind of tube very good results were obtained.

Momentary cathode rays may be caused in an ordinary incandescent lamp by connecting the filament to one pole, and a piece of tin foil, held by rubber bands to the outer or upper surface of the tube to the pole. The vacuum in this lamp, however, is too low and the cathode rays obtained do not excite X rays. Therefore the experiment, though novel, is not of any practical value.

TUBE CONNECTIONS.

The tube is connected to the secondary terminals of the spark coil as shown in the following illustration. The positive wire goes to the cathode electrode of the tube and the negative to the anode.

THE TUBE PRACTICALLY CONSIDERED.

Having provided ourselves with a suitable source of electricity, a spark coil of about 6 inches sparking distance, and a focus tube, we can connect the three as follows: If you have selected a storage battery, which may be one of three cells, giving a potential of six volts, you connect the positive and negative poles to the binding posts of the primary coil.

If you use a primary battery the cells will be equal to about one volt. You would require eight cells connected in series, as already described under the division of chemical electricity—obtaining about eight volts potential in this way.

The two open battery wires, positive and negative, are connected to the positive and negative wire with No. 18 B.W. G. gutta-percha-covered wire to the primary coil. If the connections are correct and properly made the coil is ready for use. Should it not work at once it is necessary to start the rheotome with a slight touch of the finger.

The rheotome has two purposes to accomplish. One is, that it shortens the gap in which the spring vibrates, by being pressed against it, causing it to vibrate more rapidly than when further away from it.

The points can be made of short pieces of platinum wire about $\frac{1}{8}$ inch thick, and should project $\frac{3}{16}$ of an inch over all. Do not allow the piece to be soldered to the spring, as it may thus become heated and be melted off.

In starting the rheotome with your hand there is no danger, but you should keep your hands as far away as possible from the secondary coil. The primary circuit is very small, hardly to be felt, but the secondary, as you have read, has been multiplied enormously, and is not only dangerous, but a shock resulting from it may be fatal.

The sight of a person shocked, even slightly, is an appalling scene, and the owner of the apparatus would feel much inclined to let the terrible machine alone after witnessing a shock. It is a habit of a great many operators to go carelessly about handling the wires, often receiving a shock from one wire, which is not severe; they get used to it and become negligent, but negligence must be laid aside, as a shock from the secondary or both wires may be a very serious matter.

With the vibrations of the rheotome sparks are seen to pass between the secondary dischargers. It is advisable to have a switch placed in your primary circuit, facilitating the breaking and making of the current. No. 32 B. W. G. silk-covered wire is connected to each of the secondary terminals and to the poles of the tube, as described in the former illustration, táking care not to rupture the little rings at the end of the tube. This may be avoided by bending a piece of bare copper wire or leaden fuse into the shape of a ring, into which the terminals from the secondary can be hooked; or the secondary wire may be turned upon a pencil, for several turns, removing the pencil and leaving a spring-like form which has lese tendency to injure the rings than a straight wire would.

As the current is now turned on, and all having been properly carried out as directed, a peculiar green fluorescence of the glass of the tube will be noted.

The tube should have been previously rubbed dry of all moisture with a piece of silk before connecting to the secondary coil. If the day is damp it is best to gently heat it with the flame of a spirit lamp, care being taken not to heat at one place too much at a time, and cracking the glass. When the tube is warm it may be again rubbed with a silk handkerchief. Above all means see that the wires coming from the secondary coil do not touch any part of the tube, as sparking will result and fracture of the tube follow.

When using a focus tube only half of the tube will be dark. The portion below the anode plate should be bright. If the vacuum is low, there will be a violet blue; if very low, reddish; and if broken, the sparks will pass from one electrode to the other in rapid succession.

If this green fluorescence is observed the tube is good and sending out X rays. To determine whether you have connected the tube properly, note the position of the shadow in the tube. If it is above the platinum disk, and the fluorescence is thrown downward on the greater curvature of the tube, it is connected correctly.

If the dark area is below the angle of the anode and there appears a general diffusion of the fluorescence from that pole, it will at once convince you of the fact that the tube is not properly connected. Remember the principles of the tube—that is, the focus tube, and its use, and you will make no mistake. However, testing paper, as already described, can be used. It should never be held in the hand while testing, but wound upon a glass or wooden rod and then brought in contact with the wires. Once knowing the poles of your coil you will not forget them, especially when marked as described in secondary batteries.

If, perchance, a wire ring should break at the end of the tube, it is not always necessary to throw the tube away or lay it aside to be fixed; it can be repaired temporarily by taking a little cap or loop of wire, laying it in contact with the broken end of the electrode, and fastening it down with a little sealing wax, previously heated and kneaded with the finger. The tubes so mended can be used at once with a little care.

SOURCE OF THE X RAY.[46]

The source of the ray has created a question which many have tried to solve. Roentgen, himself, was puzzled as to what it was and might be, and being of a modest disposition, instead of calling it the Roentgen ray, as it should have been termed, called it the X ray, using the algebraic term for an unknown quality or quantity.

The early experimenters in working with vacuum tubes, as has been described, believed the fluorescence to be due to an electrical action, or what not, around the cathodo pole, as has been described.

The straight lines or streams of light seemed to come from the cathode pole. You noted that, by applying a magnet to the exterior of the tube, the stream, or cathode ray, would be deviated or drawn toward the magnet; all this confirmed the fact that these rays were cathodic.

Crookes' reasons for calling it such are given in his theory of molecular bombardment, which proceeded from the cathode.

In the tubes of high vacuum, this stream or ray caused a fluorescence of the glass walls of the tube, which he believed to be due to the high molecular bombardment of the residual gas particles.

Fluorescence was again not entirely diffused, but was concentrated to a point, by the use of a concave cathode mirror or disk, which has been termed the fluorescent spot, and that the concentrated rays had the power to heat the glass to such an extent to pierce it, etc.

---

46 Interesting papers on this subject as a whole will be found in Lodge: "The rays are most powerful when the anode is struck by the cathode rays," The Elect., London, April 10, 1896; De Heen: "The anode believed to be the source of the rays," Comtes Rendus, Feb. 17, 1896; Stine: "Experiments to determine the source of X rays by making radiograms of short tube sections," Elect. World, New York, April 11, 1896.

Hertz was the first to even doubt that these rays existed externally as well as internally, and Lenard followed in his lines of theory, found them outside of the tube, but did not know that he was dealing with anything else than cathode rays.

To prevent a false conception of the terms X rays and cathode rays, we will refer to the cathode rays as those existing within the tube and the X rays as those without.

Careful study of Roentgen's reports will make these points clear to the reader.

The X rays are invisible—no human eye can perceive them. Roentgen's theory is, that the X rays are a form of longitudinal waves of ethereal vibrations, like the waves of ordinary light, but of much longer duration and length.

Others believe that X rays are just the reverse, and Tesla shares in the belief that they are streams of electrified particles thrown from that area of glass, bombarded internally by the cathode stream.

To determine whether they exist inside as well as outside of the tube, photographic plates wrapped in light proof paper have been introduced within the tube. These were not affected.[47] Another experimenter claimed that the photographic plate was not affected in vacua, and that a certain amount of atmospheric moisture was necessary. Another scientist claimed that if these X rays moved in straight lines the object struck by them would leave a well-defined shadow.

Wave motion of the ray is transmitted from one part to another. Wave length is said to be about .357 to .007 of an inch in length.

There are a number of theories and experiments recorded, but as yet nothing definite is claimed. Let us rest satisfied with the fact that the rays exist outside of

---

47 Battelli: "The X Rays Within the Vacuum Tube," Nuovo Cimento, April, 1896; Elect. Review, London, June 12, 1896.

the tube; that they cannot be reflected, except to a very slight extent—.001 degree of reflection at an incident angle of 45 degrees;[48] that the rays cannot be concentrated as yet; that they are not acted upon by a magnet,[49] but proceed from that portion of glass directly opposite the cathode pole, and are strongest at that place, although plates exposed to all sides of the tube will be more or less affected—undoubtedly by diffuse radiation originating at a point opposite the cathode.

That the X rays cannot be focused, and that all bodies are more or less pervious or transparent to them, according to their density and composition, and that they will affect a photographic plate, leaving certain shadows.

Those of greatest interest to us are the shadows of bone and softer tissue. Another important phenomenon is that certain chemicals or metallic salts fluoresce in the course of the ray.

The metallic salt used by Roentgen was the barium-platinum cyanide, but a number of these fluorescing substances have been found and are described fully in the next chapter.

REMARKS PURPORTING TO THE INDIVIDUALITY OF THE TUBE.

Select a vacuum tube according to the size of the apparatus you have, that is, if your coil gives a spark of two inches, take a tube that has its external electrodes at least three inches apart. Another important item which must be remembered is that the higher the degree of vacuum the greater is the resistance which the current has to overcome. It is necessary, therefore, to select or buy tubes that are most suitable for your special apparatus.

---

48 Rood: "Percentage of Reflection of X Rays," Science, March 27, 1896.

49 Sella & Majorana, Ecl. El., No. 10.

The tubes now made are graduated in spark lengths—as noted by the discharge from Rhumkorff coils at certain spark distances, *i.e.*, 2, 4, and 6-inch spark tubes. It would not do to buy a 6-inch spark vacuum tube for a 2-inch spark coil, as the resistance offered by the vacuum would be too great, with a result of the spark trying to jump from one electrode to the other on the outside of the tube. Another fact is that the vacuum of the tube is greatly increased by use in the secondary circuit of a coil, especially when the potentials are high enough to heat the platinum. Platinum upon cooling seems to take up more or less residual air.

A tube will work exceedingly well one day and then may have to be laid aside for several days. Experience alone will instruct the operator when his tube is working well or not and what amount of current is necessary for the making of a radiograph.

Instantaneous exposure is his goal, and if he nourishes that idea he will soon learn the idiosyncrasies of the tube. The fluoroscope, however, will help him considerably.

There is a time when the tube will no longer allow the current to pass, but remains dark or has become black on its inner walls. This indicates the high vacuum mark which your coil cannot overcome, therefore the vacuum of the tube must be lowered. This can be done by gradually heating the tube with the flame of a spirit lamp, until it is quite hot. Then connect it again to the coil and allow the current to cross through the tube; if the fluorescence does not appear, keep on heating the tube until you get the proper result.

Care must be taken to turn off the current while the tube is being heated, as a spark may pass into the alcohol receptacle, igniting the spirit, and a miniature explosion may follow, ruining the tube and lamp, not to speak of the danger to which the operator himself is subjected. Or again, the metal tube holding the wicking may draw a spark across the tube, so cracking it.

Another method to lower a high vacuum is to place the tube into a dish containing oil and boiling it in such a way upon a stove for half an hour or more.

Or it may be laid upon a piece of wood, placed in a bake oven, and heated until the glass is very hot, then gradually allowed to cool. If by placing it in circuit it has not improved, the heating may be repeated until successful. The last means of all is to have it retubed—to have it opened, the air let in and again exhausted by the vacuum pump until it gives off the rays so much desired.

The advantage of the "Standard" focus tube can be readily seen—the cathode end on the opposite side to the one having been used may be connected with the latter and put in circuit, with the result of heating. A part of the platinum anode is disintegrated in this way, and deposited in minute subdivisions upon the walls of the tube, absorbing more or less residual gas.

A tube may also be low in vacuum and still become serviceable. This is clearly brought out by Tesla as follows: He took a tube of very low vacuum and attached it to the secondary terminals of the disruptive coil. After a few minutes the color within the tube changed to an opalescent white, then to red, when the electrodes became very hot and the electro-motive force had to be reduced to prevent destruction of the electrodes. This was done by approximating the dischargers of the secondary coil to a space of an inch or more, as was deemed necessary, to bring the tube to activity.

The red color soon faded away and a white took its place, which gradually disappeared with the appearance of a fluorescent spot, which gradually grew higher and lighter, while the electrodes cooled. Then X rays were given off, no pump having been used whatever.

This same method can be resorted to when the Rhumkorff coil is used. Commence the discharge to the tube with the spark gap or terminals about one inch apart. Allow the current to pass until the electrodes heat or when the sparks commence to jump across the gap. Switch off the current, increase the distance between the spark terminals and again charge the tube. Proceed in this way until the fluorescence is of an apple-green color, or when the X rays brighten up the screen at the required distance and to the required intensity.

Care must be taken not to heat the glass too much—so preventing the piercing of the tube or its glass walls. Do not let the electrodes get above a red heat, as the disintegration of the platinum will impair the tube's vacuum. Better rest the tube at short intervals until the required effect is reached.

It has been found by Edison, and later by Tesla, who stated that a tube cooled by cold oil gave remarkable results. The bones of the hand were readily observed through a sheet of copper, iron or brass one-fourth of an inch thick. The oil was cooled in a jacket-cylinder containing cracked ice.

The latter experiments were made with a tube having only one electrode and connected to the terminals of the disruptive current transformer of Tesla.

CHAPTER V.

THE FLUOROSCOPE.

THE original fluoroscope of Roentgen consisted of a piece of paper, upon which a careless student had traced the letter A with a solution of barium-platinum cyanide, and which was later replaced by a sheet of paper coated with that salt.

Roentgen observed that the paper coated with the metallic salt and held in the X emanations became fluorescent, and that by interposing an opaque object between the tube and the screen certain shadows resulted of a degree corresponding to the density of the object held before it.

Paper, cardboard, mica and aluminium cast but little shadow. A book even of 1,000 pages impeded the fluorescence only to a slight extent. (See Roentgen's report.) But the most interesting of all shadows were those of the bones of his living hand when held before the screen. This was the first fluorescent screen used in conjunction with the X rays, although Lenard has used a similar one for determining the fluorescent value of the cathode rays, as he thought them, which without doubt must have been X rays.

Cryptoscope, iristoscope and fluoroscope are synonymous names for this screen. Professor Salvini,[50] of Rome, Italy, devised the apparatus which he called a cryptoscope. It

50 A paper read by Prof. Salvini before the Rome Med. Soc., Feb. 8, 1896; Proceedings of the Academia Medico Chirurgica di Perugia, vol. iii., Nos. 1–2; Scientific American, March 28, 1896.

consisted of a cylinder of black cardboard, closed at its lower end by a disk of the same material. The interior of this was coated with barium platinum cyanide crystals mounted upon a piece of linen with flexible collodion. At the other end of the tube a single lens was fixed for the eye. By holding this instrument in the rays a glowing or fluorescence of the salt at once appeared, lighting the interior of the cylinder, and by placing the hand upon the outer and lower end, between tube and screen, the bones of the hand could be readily seen.

Thomas Edison[51] examined the comparative fluorescent qualities of over 1,800 chemicals, and found that calcic tungstate fluoresced with six times the luminosity of barium-platinum cyanide. Next to the former was strontic tungstate. Salicylate of ammonium crystals equaled the double cyanide of potassium and barium, but differed from it in that the fluorescence increased with the thickness of the crystal layer up to one-fourth of an inch.

The following list includes the substances that fluoresce more or less under the action of the rays: Mercurious chloride, mercury diphenyl, cadmic iodide, calcic sulphide, potassic bromide, plumbic tetrametaphosphate, potassic iodide, plumbic bromide, plumbic sulphate, fluorite, powdered lead glass, pectolite, sodic cressotinate, ammonic salicylate, and salicylic acid.

The following fluoresced less: Powdered German glass, boric, calcic and sodic fluorides, sodic, mercuric, cadmic, argentic and plumbic chlorides, plumbic iodide, sodic bromide, cadmic and cadmium, lithia bromide, mercury, cadmium sulphate, uranic sulphate, phosphate, nitrate and acetate, molybdic acid, dry potassic silicate, sodic bromide, wulfenite, orthoclase, andalusite, herdinite, pyromorphite, apatite, calcite, daubusnite, calcic carbonate,

51 Elect. Review, New York, April 19, 1896.

strontic acetate, sodic tartrate, basic sulphobenzoic, calcic iodide, and natural and artificial ammonium benzoic.

A new and powerful fluorescent is the double fluoride of ammonium and uranium, discovered by Dr. Meecklebeke, of Antwerp. It is both cheap and easily made, and mounted like calcium tungstate.[52]

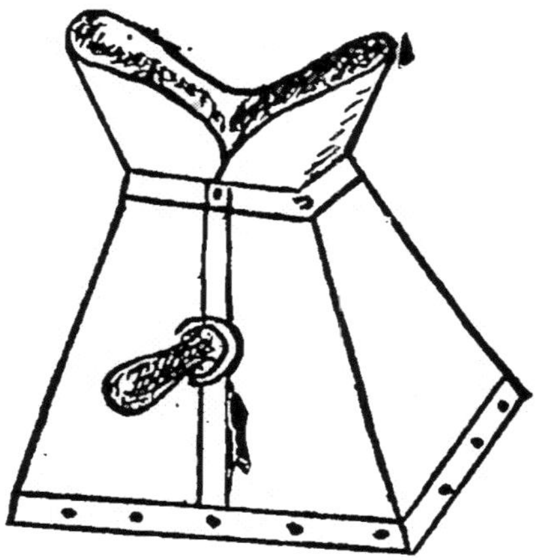

FIG. 39.

Edison designed an apparatus in which the calcic tungstate salt is used. The eyepiece has no lens but remains entirely open and shaped to accommodate both eyes. This he called the fluoroscope. (Fig. 39.)

The fluoroscope becomes at once a necessary and most valuable adjunct to radiography. Its qualities may be tabulated as follows:

1. Its simplicity of construction.
2. It enables the operator to examine the tube efficiently.
3. It enables us to study scattering radiance.
4. It enables us to obtain the detailed shadows of any opaque matter.
5. It can be readily applied to surgical diagnosis.

52 Bertrand, Medical Record, New York, January, 1897; Scientific American, Jan. 23, 1897; Kolle, Elect. Eng., Feb. 10, 1897: Elect Review, London, vol. xl.

6. It is much cheaper than the barium-platino-cyanide screen and can be readily bought or made.

1. The fluoroscope is a very simple instrument, and can be made by any one with a few pieces of heavy cardboard and the necessary amount of calcium.

2. If brought within the hemisphere of radiation, it will at once light up with a fluorescent light, enabling us to determine the amount of X-ray discharge, which, if strong, will make it exceedingly bright. This action is due to the absorption of the X rays by the chemical compound of the screen converting them to ordinary light.

3. If any opaque body be placed in front of the screen, a shadow of light and dark areas will appear upon the surface of the fluorescent screen, corresponding to the transparency or perviousness of the object when subjected to the rays.

The hand, if held in front of the fluoroscope, will cast a light outline of the fleshy parts, whereas the shadows made by the bones will be much darker.

4. The fluoroscope can be used as a means of diagnosis in determining foreign bodies in flesh or bone. Metal being more opaque than bone consequently gives a darker shadow; so that bullets, nails, pieces of steel, glass, etc., could be shown to be located in bone as well as in softer tissues.

5. Its cheapness is another factor. Barium-platino-cyanide costs considerable, a good screen made with this salt costing as much as $15.00 to $20.00 or more, whereas an 8×10-inch screen coated with the calcic salt should cost no more than $4.00.

If the reader wishes to prepare the tungstate of calcium, he can readily do so by following the instructions given below.[53]

---

53 Ogden, Scientific American.

Mix about one ounce each of chloride of sodium (common salt), tungstate of soda and chloride of calcium. The last two articles should be bought for about two cents an ounce.

Put the above ingredients, when reduced to a gross powder, into a common crucible. The author has used a fire-clay crucible with best result, costing about ten cents, to which a cover of tin must be fitted. This is placed into a glaring coal fire with coals heaped around it. Leave it remain for two or three hours, or until the contents are fused to a clear liquid. The crucible should then be taken out of the fire and set away to cool and crystallize. When cold the crucible may be broken, as it is difficult to get out the glass-like mass otherwise, then break the contents into a very coarse powder and throw it into a jar of water. The water will gradually dissolve the chloride of soda formed, and fine crystals of calcium tungstate will settle at the bottom. Remove the water above the sediment occasionally by decantation, using a rubber tube in the form of a siphon. Add clear water and allow the mixture to again settle. Decant as before and repeat until all taste of salt is gone. This usually takes about twenty-four hours of repeated washing. Pour the sediments upon heavy blotting or filtering paper and dry in sunlight.

When dry the sediment can be mounted upon a piece of tracing or linen cloth, by coating the latter with a good coat of flexible collodion—obtainable of any druggist. Common glue will answer.

Sift the fine crystalline powder upon the screen, being careful to spread it evenly all over. It is best to repeat this a second or third time when the former coating has become dry. A thickly coated screen gives much better results.

An excellent little instrument to use with the fluoroscope is the radiometer,[54] invented by the author. It consists of a small mahogany frame grooved to contain eight sections of sheet aluminium, ranging from 1 to 12 mm. in thickness. The sections have a consecutive number of holes drilled into them filled with plugs of No. 8 lead wire in such a way that No. 1, representing a section one millimeter thick, being held in front of the fluoroscope and exposed to the ray emanations, will appear as a light area of certain dimensions and containing a black spot in its center.

As the potential or tube efficiency is increased, one section after another would become more or less transparent, all showing the dark spots in the number corresponding to the plugs. The dots may be replaced with small figures of lead with little trouble.

The instrument can be readily made by any one and can be adapted to suit the operator and apparatus.

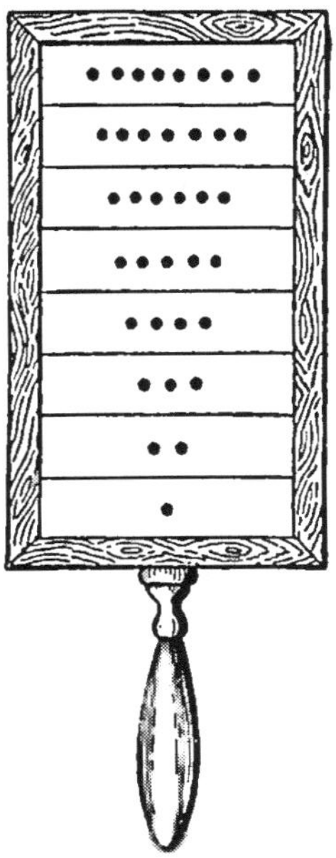

FIG. 40.

54 Kolle: "Radiometer," Elect. Eng., Dec. 9, 1896; Elect., London, August, 1897.

CHAPTER VI.

THE MODUS OPERANDI OF RADIOGRAPHY.

THE electric apparatus, the tube and its adjuncts, have been fully described, and it is now necessary to combine the whole in a proper manner to produce a radiograph.

A general description of connections of battery and coil, etc., has been given; but to fully demonstrate the complete apparatus and its relation to the subject to be radiographed, the following diagrams are given.

The source of electricity and its divisions has been dealt with. We find two of these divisions most suitable for X-ray work—namely, the battery and the dynamo.

The first are divided into closed circuit and secondary or storage batteries, and the second into alternating and direct dynamo currents.

Of all the most suitable and economical is the direct electric light current of 110 or 250 volts. The method of tapping lead wires from a socket has been shown and we will not stop to describe that again.

Having found the negative and positive wires, it is necessary to reduce the initial or street current to a lower voltage or electro-motive force, to make it suitable for the primary coil. To do this a rheostat is necessary. This can be readily obtained of an electrician. It should have at least six to eight steps, reducing the current to a known maximum and minimum, and wound to a known resistance and to a certain amperage, depending entirely upon the size of the coil used. The description of such an instrument would require considerable space, and cannot therefore be taken up. The necessary instrument can be obtained, at a very nominal price, at any electric supply house.

The connection between the rheostat and coil are made as shown in the following figure. (Fig 41.)

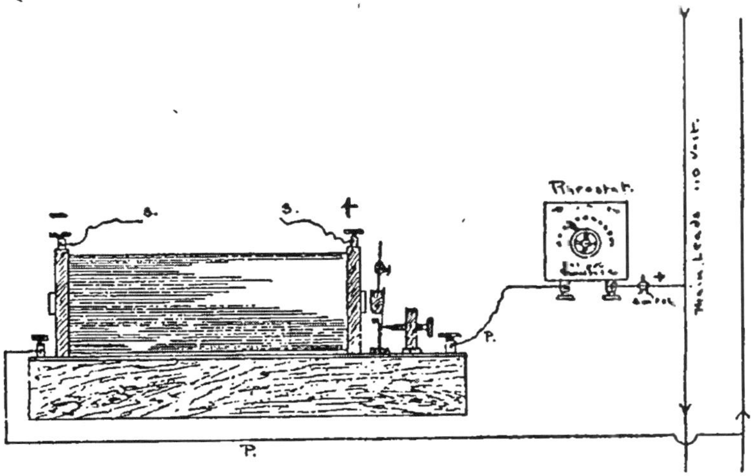

FIG. 41.

As a substitute for the rheostat a bank of incandescent lamps, as described in the chapter on Secondary Batteries, can be used.

If you are using a large coil giving from a 10 to a 14-inch spark in air, it becomes necessary to use the make-and-break wheel described in Chapter III. The connections for same are as follows: (Fig. 42.)

The positive wire is led to the one brush of the make-and break wheel, and the other attached to the remaining brush and led to the primary coil. A branch wire from each goes to the condenser of the coil, which is readily connected in the modern coils, both ending in binding posts, placed upon the coil base.

The rheostat reduces the current taken from the positive wire at 110 volts or more, and directs it to the make-and-break wheel, necessary for the primary circuit of the coil. The motor running the circuit breaker is supplied by a second lead from the street circuit. They are usually wound for 110 volts and can be connected directly to the street current of that capacity unless it is desired to regulate its speed, when the rheostat must be placed in circuit, as shown in the illustration.

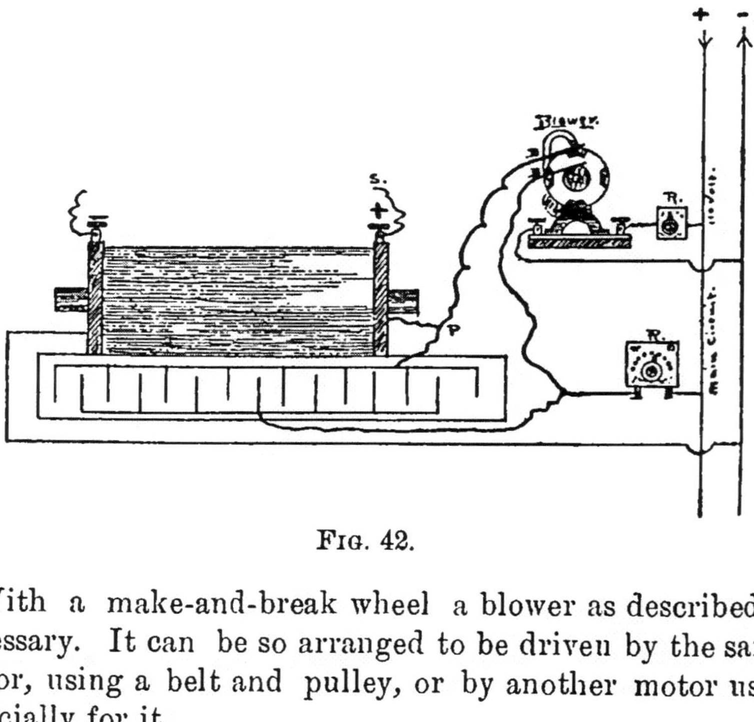

FIG. 42.

With a make-and-break wheel a blower as described is necessary. It can be so arranged to be driven by the same motor, using a belt and pulley, or by another motor used especially for it.

The make-and-break wheel suggested by Thomas Edison, is very practicable, being not only a combination of blower and circuit breaker, but allows of 8,000 to 40,000 makes and breaks per minute.

The only objection to this brass cog-wheel apparatus is the noise made while running. This is entirely overcome by that of Willyoung, of Philadelphia, which consists of an insulated or immersed break-wheel, in a cylinder containing oil or some liquid dielectric. It is also run by a motor.

It is advisable to include a switch in the main and primary circuit, so as to be able to cut it or turn off the current at will, without the danger of disconnecting wires, short circuiting, etc.

Early during my work with the Roentgen rays I became aware of the necessity of a better switching device than that used up to quite recent times; especially do I refer to the apparatus which we term a make-and-break motor. In this arrangement we have two distinct currents, the one usually of 110 volts, to run the motor proper, while another, usually a second lead from the direct main, cut down by the introduction of resistance or preferably by a suitable rheostat, goes to the make-and-break arrangement of the motor, supplying the primary of the inductive coil with a rapidly interrupted current, which has been, up to the present day, deemed highly necessary for producing the proper excitation of the necessarily high induced current of the secondary coil.

It has often happened to men, experimenting, and even to those who are quite familiar with the work, to forget to cut down the current to the rheotome or primary coil, and in consequence of the overlapping of the brushes, usually arranged on the periphery of a revolving disk, the full current has been thrown into the coil by closing down one of two switches. Although we know it is necessary to start the motor first, many a busy skiagrapher has pulled the wrong switch, sometimes to his dismay at the results, and oftener to the loss of a valuable picture.

To overcome the necessity of two switches and the other difficulties, I have devised the switch herewith shown, early last February. It is simply a double knife-switch with raised posts nearest the hinge. The rear switch is connected with the current wires of the motor, and by being closed down to the unusually high posts throws in the high volt current, starting the motor. With a second pressure the front blades are closed down, which control the lesser current intended for the primary coil.

Inasmuch as it is necessary to shut down the current to the primary first, all that is required is to raise the switch partly, so cutting off that current. It can again be closed, with the motor running at full speed as desired. By pulling up the switch entirely, both currents are cut off, stopping both.

It is a neat little device and should be added to every

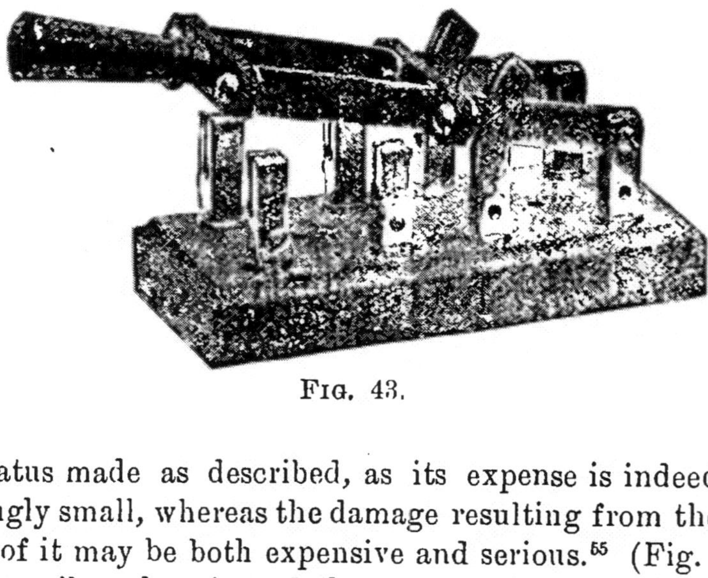

FIG. 43.

apparatus made as described, as its expense is indeed exceedingly small, whereas the damage resulting from the absence of it may be both expensive and serious.[55] (Fig. 43.)

Never allow the wires of the main or branch of one to come in contact, as an unpleasant sparking will occur, and the fuse in circuit will be blown at once, leaving the operator in total darkness.

The tube is connected to the secondary terminals. The reader cannot study the chapter on vacuum tubes too carefully, as considerable trouble must be expected at first.

55 Kolle: "Switch for X Ray Work," Elect. Eng., Dec. 9, 1897.

He should be prepared to grasp the cause of difficulties without delay. If there is a question in doubt, it will be found advisable to refer to that chapter until the operator becomes acquainted with the pros and cons of the tube and its irregularities.

With the tube connected, we find ourselves at a loss as to how to fasten the tubes in a more desirable position than by hanging it from the terminals of the coil. For this means a light wooden laboratory stand with a heavy base is most suitable. The clamp of the tube holder should contain a piece of cork on either side, or should be ribbed to engage a cork slipped over the elongated portion of the tube, made for that purpose.

Another source of current is that from a battery of cells. A number of these have been described and the necessary number of cells is usually from eight to sixteen, connected in series to the primary coil. The rheotome is most suitable as a circuit breaker, in this case, unless the means of running the motor make-and-break wheel can be obtained. The connections are made as already described.

If a secondary battery is used it is always advisable to interpose a resistance into the circuit, as it sometimes happens that the plugs of platinum of the rheotome fuse, in that event short-circuiting the coil, possibly injuring its insulation, buckling the battery cells, and destroying them by so rapid a discharge.

The size of the battery depends upon the size of the coil used. Knowing that each cell gives about 2 volts, it becomes necessary to connect several in series to make up the primary circuit.

For a 6-inch coil a battery of 4 to 6 cells is necessary, and for a 10 to 12-inch coil 8 to 10 cells are required. A good storage battery of small and portable size is that made by the Chloride Accumulator Company, which answers the purpose very well. The capacity of discharge should be at least 30 amperes per hour. The cells should never be discharged under 1.7 volts, and ought to be recharged at least once in five weeks. To test the voltage of the primary battery, the volt meter is required; but the operator could provide himself with a set of testing lamps, ranging from 1.5 to 12 volts, used as follows: When a 2-volt lamp, placed in circuit with the battery, refused to give a bright light the discharge should be discontinued and the battery recharged.

For making exposures of patients when placed upon a

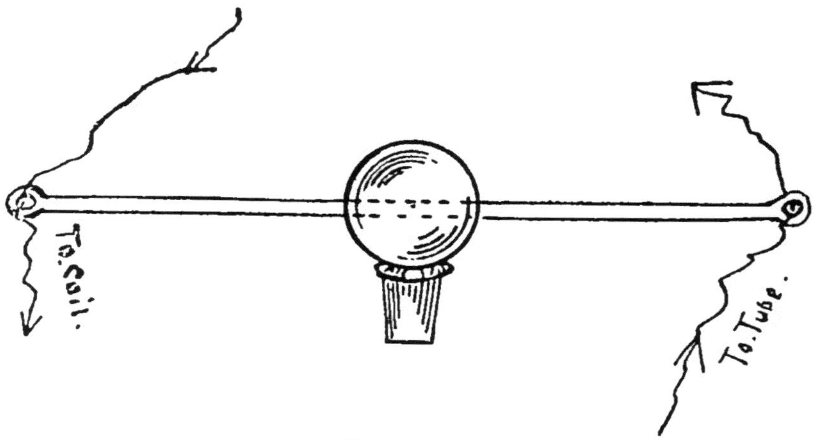

Fig. 44.

table or within a bed, a large laboratory stand is required. It should have an iron base to prevent jostling or upsetting.

The author has found difficulty in the early experiments in holding the wires going to the tube in a good position and has added a little device for holding them in place, which can be attached to any of these wooden laboratory stands. (Fig. 44.)

It consists of a divided sphere or ball of wood, having a lower wedge-shaped projection made to fit into a hole made in the stand proper, and a longitudinal groove in either half, lined with cork, to accommodate a rod of wood or glass.

The latter should have two eyelets or hooks at each end to engage the wires. Rods for the purpose can be readily made by heating the ends of a glass tube to a white heat and bending it into the required shape with a dressing forceps.

The wires should be about four inches further apart than the sparking distance of the coil.

The plug slightly moistened is inserted into the opening made in the stand. Terminal wires can be passed through the eyelets or either end of this holder and connected to the vacuum tube. Another advantage of this little addition is to keep the wires away from the sides of the tube and also allows of a better contact when rings are used as terminals for the vacuum tube.

With the tube in position the current is turned on. If your apparatus is not provided with the Kolle switch, begin by closing the switch to the motor or blower, if you are using this, and regulate its speed by the rheostat, placed in circuit for that purpose.

The current to the coil is then turned on, being sure that the rheostat handle is brought down to its last step or that its highest resistance is thrown into the circuit. At once the tube will begin to show signs of fluorescence or activity.

If the fluorescence is not quite bright enough, or the fluoroscope does not become as highly fluorescent as is necessary, the handle of the rheostat must be turned one step forward and advanced as is necessary, noted by the results obtained in the tube, etc.

Now you take up the most useful of all divisions in this work, namely, the fluoroscope, which shows the value of the X ray emanations by their power of causing fluorescence of the screen of that instrument. If the crystals appear dark and murky, advance the handle of the rheostat one more step. Again inspect the rays with the fluoroscope, and if quite bright, hold your hand in front of its base, or between the tube and the fluoroscope, and you will at once notice that the bones appear as dark shadows upon the screen, while the flesh of the hand falls away, as it were, and is shown by a lighter outline or shading.

If you put in still less resistance, the flesh shadow recedes still more, and the bones appear as naked, resembling the articulated hand of the bony skeleton. When such a result appears upon the screen you have the proper X rays, and of enough power to make an excellent radiograph of the hand or other object. Switch off the current to the coil, and if necessary the make-and-break wheel motor current, and go to your dark room. This must be placed at a good distance—at least 40 to 60 feet away; or, better still, have it in another floor entirely from that upon which the apparatus is, as clouding of the photographic plates by the rays is sure to occur within a shorter distance. Place the plate to be used into its holder. Be sure that that is light proof and take it into the operating room. Lay it film side up, with the object placed directly upon the plate or film side as contained in the holder.

If an ordinary plate holder is used, an ebonite or aluminium slide should take the place of the rubber one. It is not necessary to remove the slide to make a radiograph. The object is directly laid upon it.

The distance of the plate and object from the tube varies with the density of the object and the power of the rays given off by the tube used. It has been found that a limited distance gives a better picture, with well-defined outline. Experience can therefore be the best guide to the operator. A small object of little opacity or density can be placed at a greater distance when a good tube and a large coil is employed than *vice versa*.

For the hand a distance of from 4 to 12 inches, for the tube from the plate, may be found necessary when using a coil giving from a 2 to a 6-inch spark discharge. If, for example, you wish to make a radiograph of the hand, and your coil gives a spark of 6 inches with a powerful fluorescence of the screen, and a good skiograph or fluorograph of the hand is observed upon the screen, you would have to place the hand upon the plate as mentioned, and placed at a distance of from 12 to 18 inches, or even more, to get a good sharp outline.

With smaller coils and less powerful rays the distance between the tube and plate must naturally be reduced. Remember that the nearer you bring the object to the tube the more powerful is the action of the rays and *vice versa*. A plate exposed at a distance of 6 inches will have to be exposed nine times as long as at a distance of 2 inches.

The object, as before said, is laid upon the plate holder, containing the plate to be exposed. The current is turned on to the already regulated motor and to the make-and-break wheel. A few necessary instructions must be given to the patient, or person sitting, to prepare him for the work.

A few minutes of explanation sometimes saves a number of plates, as the uninstructed will naturally start at the snapping and buzzing of the coil and its adjuncts, and also by the unexpected fluorescence of the tube. It is best to tell them what to expect before the apparatus is brought into action. If the patient is a child it is advisable to go through the entire operation, showing the child the coil and the tube in action. Within a few minutes it will become accustomed to the procedure, enabling you to secure a good negative by a short exposure, without constant movement on the part of the patient. It may be necessary to hold the arm or limb to be radiographed so to prevent their moving during the exposure.[56]

An expert using a 10-inch spark coil can make a picture

56 See Kolle, an appliance for securing proper radiographs about the elbow joint. Elect. Eng., March 31, 1897.

of the hand and forearm in 4 to 8 seconds, at a distance of 18 to 26 inches. The amateur should give enough time in all exposures, at least until he becomes familiarized with the apparatus and the results obtained. Remember there is less danger of over-exposure than under-exposure. The best method for determining time is to develop the negatives personally. They will show the differences of time of exposure at once in their time of developing.

An over-exposed plate is quickly developed, and turns black in a short time, whereas an under-exposed plate takes minutes and sometimes as much as an hour or more to develop.

It is best to make radiographs of a few small objects to begin with and develop the negatives yourself, to accomplish good results, and even the dexterity of an expert.

By all means study the tube effects with the fluoroscope, and when accustomed to that use the radiometer which can be graded to suit the operator or coil, furnishing at once a reliable and ever-ready means of telling the distance for, and necessary time of, exposure.

Some experimenters claim that by inserting a spark gap in the secondary circuit, efficiency of the tube would be increased, and that better results can be obtained from low vacuum than in circuits where the spark gap is not employed. This gap should be inserted at the positive or anode pole, and its width regulated according to the effects produced in the tube.

When making a long exposure, say from 20 to 30 minutes, it is advisable to rest the tube from time to time, as best results are obtained from a cool or cold vacuum tube with cold electrodes, as already shown. A platinum disk heated to a white heat may give good results, but it is advisable to allow the disks to remain below that point, as the tube would soon be rendered low in vacuum by the disintegration of its metallic composition.

When the object has been exposed for a given time, the currents of the motor and coil are turned off, and the plate is removed to the dark room ready to be developed, etc.

If a radiogram of a foreign body is to be made, *i.e.*, a bullet in the limb, where its exact location is required, two plates or negatives must be made. One laterally, giving the lateral view of the part and the depth of the foreign body contained within, and the other negative directly antero-posterior, giving the distance of the foreign object from the outer borders of the limb. By comparing the two negatives, depth and distance can be exactly measured.

Another method of determining the exact location of a foreign body is obtained by triangulation.[57] For this two tubes are used, placed a slight distance apart, so that two shadows of objects are thrown upon the dry plate.

By measuring the relative position of the tubes and object radiographed upon the plate or seen upon the screen, imaginary lines may be drawn from the picture to the screen or dry plate to the tubes, which will be found to cross or bisect exactly at the position of the object to be located. The former method, however, is much simpler, readily applied and less confusing to an amateur geometrician.

If a radiograph of a limb in splints is to be made, and the latter are composed of wood or felt, they can be allowed to remain on the limb during the exposure, as well as bandages, etc. Stiff starch bandages are not opaque and need not be removed. A plaster of paris cast must, however, be removed, to obtain pictures of the bones, etc.

Bandages are not opaque and, as has been said, need not be removed; in fact, you may find it necessary to bandage

---

57 See, also, Dr. N. S. Scott, "The Location, by Triangulation, of Foreign Bodies in the Hand," American X-Ray Journal, June, 1897.

the plate to the limbs of children so that they may be firmly and safely held during the time of exposure.

Shoes should be removed, although leather offers but little obstruction—yet the eyelets, buttons and nails in the heel and sole of the shoe would show, obliterating certain portions of the bony structure.

The object radiographed must be brought as close to the plate as possible to obtain an exact outline. It is therefore found necessary to remove extra clothing or bulging bandages.

Patients are best radiographed in bed, with the part to be exposed laid upon the plate holder. The tube employed can be fixed into the proper position by the use of the large laboratory stand described.

MANIFOLDING.

By the suggestion of Prof. Elihu Thomson,[58] manifold copies of an object may be made as follows: The X rays being very powerful in their penetrating power, more than one sheet of photographic and sensitive paper would be affected, and in such a way several impressions of an object could be made.

Sensitive bromide papers do not give as good results as films, which the author advises the reader to use. They are exceedingly thin, will give excellent negatives, and may be developed the same as dry plates.

Stereoscopic radiograms were also first suggested by Professor Thomson,[59] and found to give exceedingly beautiful contour and perspective. They can be made as follows: Expose the objects upon the one plate as usual. Then take

---

58 From "Thomson's Experiments:" Elect. Eng., New York, March 11, April 8 and 22, 1896; Elect. Review, New York, April 8, 1896.

59 "Stereoscopic Sciagraphy," Thomson: Elect. World, New York, March 14, 1896.

a second plate and expose same with the objects and tube in their relative displacement. By placing the two developed negatives into the ordinary stereoscope a very pleasing effect is obtained. The picture appears more lifelike and not flat and uncanny as in the usual proof or negative.

This method can also be used in the lantern stereoscope by making a lantern slide of the two negatives. With the aid of a newly invented lantern, it can be thrown upon the screen with an effect both striking and pleasing.

Dr. MacIntyre, of Glasgow,[60] claims he has made a radiograph in a very small fraction of a second, using a flash or a single interruption of the spark coil. He used the mercury interrupter in conjunction with an 11-inch coil. The interrupter, as said, allows of a high primary current and naturally a higher secondary induced current, giving high fluorescecne of considerable actinic power.

The reader may use the ordinary rheotome for flashing or snap-shot exposures as follows: Screw the tension screw back, so that the hammer head is a fair distance from the core or magnet, or until the usual current will not move it. Then connect up a strong primary current much stronger than usually used; and with everything in readiness—*i.e.*, the tube, plates, etc.—press the head of the hammer toward the core of the coil until a spark passes. Then develop the plate, and if not sufficiently clear, repeat the experiment, allowing this time two or more sparks to pass, etc.

Care should be taken in flashing, as it puts considerable strain on the secondary insulation, and may produce heat enough to burn the silk covering of the wires, possibly burning the wires, arcing or short-circuiting the coil. Ten successive sparks is all that will be advisable to allow to pass through the spark gap in this way with safety at any one time.

---

60 MacIntyre: Photogram, London, June, 1896, p. 156.

CHAPTER VII.

THE PHOTOGRAPHIC APPARATUS.

ALTHOUGH this century may, and very truly, be called the electric age, there are few persons who have not dabbled more or less in photography.

The knowledge of photography is of great advantage to the radiographer, although no camera or lens are used, no lights and shades have to be carefully dealt with, and yet a most important branch of that art is necessary for the production of a radiograph, radiogram or skiagraph, etc., all synonymous terms appertaining to a picture or print made of a negative produced by an exposure to the X rays.

First of all a dark room is necessary. A good-sized closet having a few shelves, a sink and running water is all that is required. Where a large room is used, the windows, if present, must be covered first with orange paper and above that with two thicknesses of black needle paper, occluding all white light. A ruby lamp is an indispensable article in a dark room. It should be of good size and burn petroleum oil.

Several sized hard rubber or glass trays are necessary, and the author advises two 8×10 and two 16×18 inches.

The dry plates or films to be used are next selected. There are a number of these upon the market, of all makes and rapidity. Some operators have used the slow or landscape plates or *vice versa* with excellent results, but I have found that any reliable plate of medium rapidity answers very well.

Rapid plates seem to give the best results, whereas the ultra-rapid dry plates of 40 sensitometer, called extra rapid or lightning plates, require very careful handling and are readily fogged by the least trace of white, or other than ruby light, and do not give any better results.

A plate of 100 to 75 sensitometer is about the best to use. Celluloid films can be employed, being much lighter and less breakable.

A proper receptacle or holder for the plate or film is also required, and I have used envelopes of orange and black needle paper, made to fit the plates, without one single failure. The envelope should be made to fit the plate or film loosely, so that it may be used over and over again. The best method of making them is to take an ordinary piece of glass of the plate size and make the envelope over this, using glue to stick the turned ends together. The orange paper is used first and the black over that. Two layers of black paper are necessary. The one end of the envelope so formed is left open for the removal and introduction of the plates, leaving enough paper at this end to turn over or to be folded over in such a way as to occlude all light when the plate is placed inside.

I have also found it advisable to gum a small disk of white paper about one-half inch in diameter on the upper side of the envelope, to indicate the film side of the plate within. This ofttimes prevents mistakes in turning the plate upside down for an exposure. When using these envelopes always place the dry plate with its film side and the little white disk on the envelope facing upward.

The ordinary plate-holder can be used, replacing its slide with an ebonite one. There is a disadvantage in these, however, in that the plate is too deeply placed within the frame, and therefore the object is not, except in the center of the plate, in close contact with the latter, giving an indistinct or foggy image of the object exposed.

I have devised a novel plate-holder that practically overcomes this difficulty. It is composed of a light-proof holder of aluminium, having a white disk mounted on its upper side as in the paper-holder. They are particularly advantageous where moist or perspiring objects are to be radiographed, *i.e.*, wet bandages or wet dressings applied to the part, and may even be used in fresh fractures where bleeding has not been thoroughly controlled. When the paper envelopes are used, it is best to lay a piece of dry cloth or several layers of blotting paper between the moist object and the plate, as the penetration of the moisture ruins the activity of the sensitive film, leaving opaque spots on the negative and often obstructing the very part which needs to be exposed by this method of radiography.

The exposed plate when developed becomes the negative. The negative is said to be exposed when the plate has been subjected to light, or in this case to the action of the X rays.

After the plate is exposed it is developed. For this purpose certain chemical compounds are necessary, known under the name of developers.

There are a considerable number of these developing solutions—in fact, every manufacturer of dry plates recommends a certain formula, but one developer usually answers for all.

I have always used the so-called "Eikonogen" developer, which is made as follows:

No. 1. Distilled water, 2,400 ccm. (80 oz.); sulphite of soda (crystals), 115 grams (3½ oz.); oxalic acid, 4 grams (1 dr.); eikonogen, 90 grams (1½ oz.); prussiate of potash (yellow), 15 grams (1 oz.). Dissolve the eikonogen in hot water and mix.

No. 2. Distilled water, 600 ccm. (20 oz.); carbonate of potash, 60 grams (2 oz.).

The two solutions (Nos. 1 and 2) should be mixed as follows to make the developer: Take 4 ounces of No. 1 and add one-half ounce of No. 2 to same. When mixed it is ready for use.

In winter the developer should be slightly warmed to about 60 or 70 degrees Fahrenheit. In summer it should be used cold. For this purpose it may be laid on ice for a few minutes, or a small piece of ice may be added to the solution in the tray.

Assuming that you have exposed a dry plate in the way described in Chapter VI., you retire to the dark room with the plate still inclosed in the light-proof holder.

To develop the plate, mix the two solutions as stated and pour into a tray large enough to hold the plate. Then remove the plate from the holder, being sure there is no other light than that which comes from the ruby lamp, and place the plate, film side up, quickly into the developer, in such a way that the entire film is immersed in the solution. Rock the tray to and fro for several minutes, when the parts most exposed to the X rays will begin to darken and blacken gradually. After a few moments the object radiographed will appear. If the hand has been exposed it will be found that the flesh outline will appear, first, as a white image lying upon a dark or black background. By further development, the flesh will be seen to fade away, leaving but an image of the bones in white color. When thus far developed, remove the plate from the solution carefully, and hold it in front of the ruby lamp. If you can look through the plate and make out all the details, the negative is sufficiently developed. If, however, the picture is not readily made out, the plate must be again placed into the developer and developed until they are quite plain.

A very good way to study the progress of a developing plate is to remove the plate from the solution from time to time, and looking at its reverse or glassy side the image will be seen on this, in white outline, when fully developed.

The image is said to be "through" when observed from the glass side of the plate. Remember that what appears white in the negative becomes black in the print or positive.

It is difficult to determine the exact time necessary for developing, as every exposure may differ; but by carrying out the directions, a plate exposed about four or five minutes ought to develop in about three minutes. However, if the developer is weak, which it should always be to save the details of the picture, as fast developers flash up the image too quickly and consequently darken them and the finer shades. A plate may require as much as 15 or 20 minutes to develop.

Do not develop too long, because the details are then obliterated and a poor positive results. This may be observed by the film of the plate turning gray or bluish gray.

If you find that the plate develops too quickly, add a little water to the developer, which will restrain its action according to the quantity added, and give a thin negative. This will print much faster than if dense, and care must be taken in printing the sensitive paper, as will be described later.

To obtain more intensity in the negatives—that is, if the negatives appear weak and too thin, add 10 grams of hydrochinon to solution No. 1.

Another good developer is the "Metol," made as follows: Distilled water, 50 oz.; metol (Hauf), ½ oz.; dissolve the metol in the water and add sulphite of soda (crystals), 5 oz.

No. 2. Pure water, 10 oz.; carbonate of potash, 1 oz.

For use take 4 ounces of No. 1 and 2 drams of No. 2. If the plate is underexposed, or slow in developing, add a little more of No. 2, or if the plate develops too quickly, a little of No. 1 solution added to the above mixture will be found to restrain its action and give an excellent negative.

With the above developer, the plate may be observed to turn uniformly black, instead of the beautiful white image given by the eikonogen or eikonogen-hydrochinon, but upon fixing a very good and soft negative results.

If you have developed the plate as described it must be taken out of the developer and thoroughly washed in clean running water for several minutes and then placed into the fixing bath, to make the image on the plate permanent. The fixing bath removes all that sensitive chemical from the gelatin film not acted upon by the rays, and prepares the negative for exposure to light and printing purposes.

The bath is composed of water, 1 gallon, and hyposulphite of sodium, 2 pounds.

The negative is laid into a second tray containing the fixing solution. The plate should be well covered by the solution. The time allowed for this process depends upon the strength of the bath or solution used. A fresh solution will fix a negative in a few minutes.

To determine whether a plate is thoroughly fixed, lift it out of the tray and hold it to the ruby light. If it appears perfectly clear without mottling and no white areas here and there, it is done and can be safely carried into another room and inspected in daylight.

The negative must then be thoroughly washed in running water for 20 minutes to remove all trace of the hypo, which is removed with difficulty from the gelatin film. I would recommend a washing tank for this purpose, made of wood and containing slanting grooves to hold the plate, which should rest on a strip of wood placed about an inch above the bottom of the tank, thus allowing a free circulation of water underneath and around the plate. The water should enter at the bottom and overflow on top. Crystallization on the negative and fading are caused by insufficient washing or uneliminated hypo.

If a number of transverse lines are seen to cross over the

film it should be replaced into the hypo bath until it is perfectly clear.

By examining the negative you will find that the image, if of the right hand, will appear as such, whereas the print obtained from the same negative would give a reversed image, as if the radiogram had originally been made of the left hand. This is due to the fact that the exposure of the plate was made with the film side near or in close contact with the object, and had to be reversed in printing, so that the film side, instead of being turned up, is now turned down toward the sensitive or printing paper, to make the positive or picture.

For washing the negative cold water should always be used, otherwise the gelatin will frill or even melt, ruining the plate. This occurs frequently in summer, when the water from the hydrant is lukewarm, and should always be guarded against by adding a piece of ice to the water in the tank or tray.

To harden the film of the negative, immerse the plate in a solution composed of one dram of burnt alum to a pint of water, for a few minutes before the final washing.

When the negative has been thoroughly washed as directed, it is placed on a rack or shelf to dry. Never put the plate near a stove to make it dry quickly, as the heat will melt the gelatin and not a trace of the much-prized picture will remain. A warm room free of dust is best for drying the negative.

It has often occurred in my practice that the surgeon or physician is anxious to obtain the negative as quickly as possible, and the slow-drying process of the film could not be used. In this case the plate must be placed in a perfectly clean tray and enough alcohol (95 per cent.) to cover the plate, poured into it. The plate can be removed after several minutes and be placed where it is exposed to a draft of air, which evaporates the alcohol and leaves a dry and hardened film, that can be safely handled in a short time. A thin overexposed negative may be placed into subdued sunlight to dry. This will darken or intensify it.

To intensify a very thin negative, which has been fixed and thoroughly washed, place it into a solution composed of water, 50 parts; bichloride of mercury, 1 part; bromide of potassium, 1 part.

When the film has become perfectly white, it has been completely bleached and is washed off, to rinse the mercury out of the film. It is then placed into a second solution, composed of equal parts of a saturated solution of sulphite of soda and water; or, concentrated ammonia, 1 dram; water, 1 pint.

Upon placing the plate into either one of the above solutions, the whitened film will slowly and steadily become darkened until the proper density is obtained. The plate is removed and again washed free of the sulphite or ammonia, and allowed to dry as before.

PRINTING.

The plate having been developed, fixed, washed and dried, is ready to use for printing.

For prints a number of sensitized papers can be found in the markets, but the albumen or collodion papers are to be preferred for this class of work. Some of these are the Solio, Kloro, Kloro-Special, Aristo, etc. I have used Kloro and Solio papers with good results.

To print or make the positive or picture, place the negative into a printing frame, film side down or rather inward toward the frame, and lay a sheet of the printing paper, with its prepared or sensitized surface in contact with the film side of the negative; close the frame by placing the spring back gently and firmly into place, closing or locking the springs provided with each frame. The closed frame, glass side up, is placed into sunlight and allowed to remain until the sensitized paper has turned to a medium purple color. It is then removed and a second one takes its place—according to the number of prints desired. Care must be taken in printing, especially when thin negatives are used, as burning of the paper results or too dark a positive will be obtained, which will obliterate the finer details. It is best to print these in subdued sunlight or under white tissue paper.

The proper tone to print to is a little darker than the color of the picture desired. The print will lose a good deal in toning, and is now ready for toning. All prints transferred from the frame should be put into a light-proof box until the required number have been made.

The prints must then be washed in several changes of water, to remove the silver, which has not been acted upon by the exposure to sunlight, and are then ready for the toning bath, of which we have two kinds, the combined and the separate. The combined bath is certainly a very useful one, as a print can be toned in very little time, compared with that of the separate bath. The difficulty with this process of toning, however, is the instability of the pictures so produced; in other words, the pictures so made are not permanent and will fade to a yellow color in several weeks. In fact, the picture may disappear altogether in time.

It is not advisable for the amateur to make his own combined bath. The separate or stock solutions are complex and the ingredients must be solved in earthenware crocks in hot water of 160 F., etc. A large quantity must be made to make its use practicable, and the results obtained do not warrant the amount of trouble involved in its preparation. There are, however, several good combined toning baths sold on the market, and I have used the "Ilo" and "N. Y. Aristo" preparations with exceedingly good results. They can be obtained at almost any photo-supply house.

The prints are immersed in the bath and toned to the desired shade, then placed into the following bath for final fixing and to clear them: Water, 1 pint; hyposulphite of soda, 1½ ounces; sodium chloride, 1 ounce; sulphite of soda (crystals), 1 dram.

They should remain in this bath about three or five minutes, and then washed for one hour in twelve or sixteen changes of water. After washing, the prints are placed upon a glass plate until the greater part of the water has drained off, leaving the paper still moist and ready to mount upon cardboard mounts, with starch paste.

The separate bath, as before said, is the more reliable of the two baths used for toning, and is made as follows:

No. 1. Water, 20 ounces; sodium acetate, 5 grains; borax (powdered), 5 grains.

No. 2. Chloride of gold (Merk), 15 grains; water, 16 ounces.

For toning take 20 ounces of No. 1 and ½ ounce of No. 2 solution. Allow the prints to remain in the bath until the desired tone is obtained and place in clean water before fixing.

The toning bath should be kept alkaline. For this purpose a saturated solution of sodium acetate can be kept at hand and added to the bath as necessary to keep the bath as required. Litmus paper is a valuable addition to the toning bath. Small strips of the alkaline and the acid papers are allowed to float around in the bath. By the change of their color the acidity or alkalidity of the bath is determined.

The prints are now ready to be fixed, and the bath for this process is made as follows: Sodium hyposulphate, 1 ounce; water, 1 pint.

This bath should be kept acid by the addition of about 2 grains of meta-bisulphate of potassium.

Twenty minutes of fixing is all that is necessary. The

prints are then removed and placed into a hardening bath, as most papers soften during the process of toning and fixing. The latter bath is composed of alum (chrome), ½ ounce to the pint of water. The latter may be combined with the fixing bath, making a hypo-alum bath, but I prefer to use them separate, as the latter is not always required.

The prints should be thoroughly washed and mounted with starch paste upon the proper mounts.

To give the picture the desired gloss after mounting they should be polished. This is best done by a photographer, as the necessary burnishers, to be good, cost considerable, and the burnishing of half a dozen large prints should not cost over twenty-five cents.

For all practical purposes the negative should be used, as that gives all the finer details which are lost more or less in printing.

To exhibit a negative, without injuring the film of the plate, it may be placed into an ordinary wood frame and covering the film side with a clean glass plate of the same size as the negative and fastening the two into the frame, as you would any transparent. In this way it may be thoroughly inspected or shown without danger to the plate.

Lantern slides are better in one respect than the print, as they retain the details. They should be made directly from the negative by a reliable firm. To make or prepare them yourself would take considerable time and necessary apparatus, and the necessary directions would require more space than practicable, therefore I would recommend the radiographer to intrust them to regular lantern slide makers. The cost per slide for making should not exceed one dollar. J. B. Colt & Co., of New York City, have made slides of all my negatives for lecturing purposes.

Now a word or two on the reduction of the time of exposure. As I have said in the earlier part of this volume, the reduction in the time of exposure necessary to procure a proper radiogram of an object, of whatever nature, is the direction in which the operator must direct his studies.

We have already made wonderful strides in this direction, as shown in the last chapter.

Early during the first months of experimentation, Professors Pupin [61] and Swinton [62] advised the use of a fluorescent screen placed in contact with the film of the dry plate, for the purpose of reducing the time of exposure.

The film of the plate, in being exposed in this way, was in reality acted upon by the light which the chemical compound of the screen emitted, brought about by its absorption of the X rays converting them into ordinary light. This is certainly an exceedingly good method and is recommended by a number of operators. The result, however, shows a granular effect of the negative, unless a finely powdered chemical is employed for the screen. I would recommend the finest crystalline powder of calcium tungstate as the best.

Tesla has used a fluorescent powder, dusted upon the film of the dry plate, with good results. However, the former method of Pupin is far more practicable, as the screen can be used over and over again without loss of material—naturally occurring in the Tesla method.

Photographic plate manufacturers have recently introduced special or X ray plates. These differ from the usual dry plate, in having some fluorescent material incorporated in the film of sensitized gelatin. The action of the X rays upon such a film will, as may readily be expected, be much more active, lessening the time of

---

61 Electricity, New York, Feb. 12, 1896.

62 Swinton: The Electrician, London, April 24, 1896; Henry, C.: Comptes Rendus, Feb. 10, 1896: "The use of phosphor—sulphide of zinc to reduce time of exposure."

exposure considerably, and giving an exceedingly good outline of the object radiographed.

The special X ray plates are manufactured by Carbutt & Co., of Philadelphia, and B. J. Edwards & Co., of London. Their cost is little more than the ordinary plate. They may be obtained in two forms, wrapped in light proof paper, ready for use, and uncovered as all other plates.

Negatives made with the special plates do not only give better pictures in details, but also good density for printing purposes.

Another method to shorten the time of exposure is to heat the ordinary plate. A warm plate or its contained silver is rendered more active or sensitive than when cold.

There are a number of other methods used in connection with the dry plate with the view of shortening the time of exposure, but I have given the more reliable ones which give the best results and are used by most all expert operators.

FLUOROPHOTOGRAPHY.

It is undoubtedly familiar to you, that whatever the eye can see can be reproduced by the camera or photographic apparatus, no matter what the object may be. We have been enabled in the past to even photograph a minute object, so small that the eye can hardly appreciate it, by the use of the microphotoscope. Again, by the combined use of mirrors, set at respective angles, the interior of living organs, such as the stomach, bladder, etc., have been photographed.

I have shown how readily an opaque object, such as the hand, can be rendered transparent to the human eye, to such a degree that the bones appear in darker shade than that of flesh, by the use of the charged tube and fluoroscope. Now if the eye can appreciate this image or picture, there is no reason why it could not be photographed. As has been shown, the chemical compound of the screen converts the X rays into ordinary light by its absorption of the rays, leaving a shadow or skiograph of the object where the rays have not entirely penetrated. An object therefore will cast a shadow according to its density or perviousness.

Dr. J. M. Bleyer,[63] of the Royal Academy of Naples, probably conceived the idea of photographing the skiograph directly from the fluorescent screen, before any other scientist. He constructed a special apparatus for this purpose, which he calls the Fluoro-photoscope. It is simply a fluoroscope, mounted upon the lens of a camera, in such a way, that the skiograph or luminous picture seen upon the screen is focused upon the ordinary dry plate and exposed as ordinarily in open air.[64]

The exposure in this experiment, to obtain a good negative, requires a little more time than when the plate is exposed to daylight. The proper time necessary would be equal to an exposure in fogged sunlight. This would be about from two to six minutes. Excellent results are obtained and the experiment may be tried by any one who is fortunate to possess both electrical apparatus and a camera.

---

63 Bleyer: Trans. Roy. Acad. Med. and Surg., Naples, April 7, 1896.

64 Elect. Eng., New York, July 1, 1896.

CHAPTER VIII.

THE NATURE OF THE RAYS.

ALTHOUGH Dr. Roentgen claims all solid bodies emit X rays to a certain extent, none show the power of rays as well as those given off from a charged vacuum tube.

A great many experimenters have tried to show that the X rays were similar in their action, when compared to the results obtained from exposures to ultra-violet rays of sunlight. But it is known that the results so obtained were merely due to infiltration of light, and not to X rays. The light in these experiments found its way through the slide or cover of the plate holder, and left but a shadow of the object as a whole.

To positively ascertain if any such phenomena as the X rays were contained in sunlight, a large lens was constructed for the purpose of making definite experiments. No different results were obtained. Plates inclosed in holders with objects laid upon them were also exposed to moonlight, and the same effect as with ordinary or concentrated sunlight was obtained.

That the X rays resemble or are greatly similar to the nature of ultra-violet light there is little doubt; in fact a number of scientists have almost accepted the theory of their kindred nature. Dr. Oliver Lodge,[65] in his summarization of the surviving hypothesis of the nature of the X rays, says that "In the remarkable discovery of MM.

65 The Electrician, London, July 17, 1896.

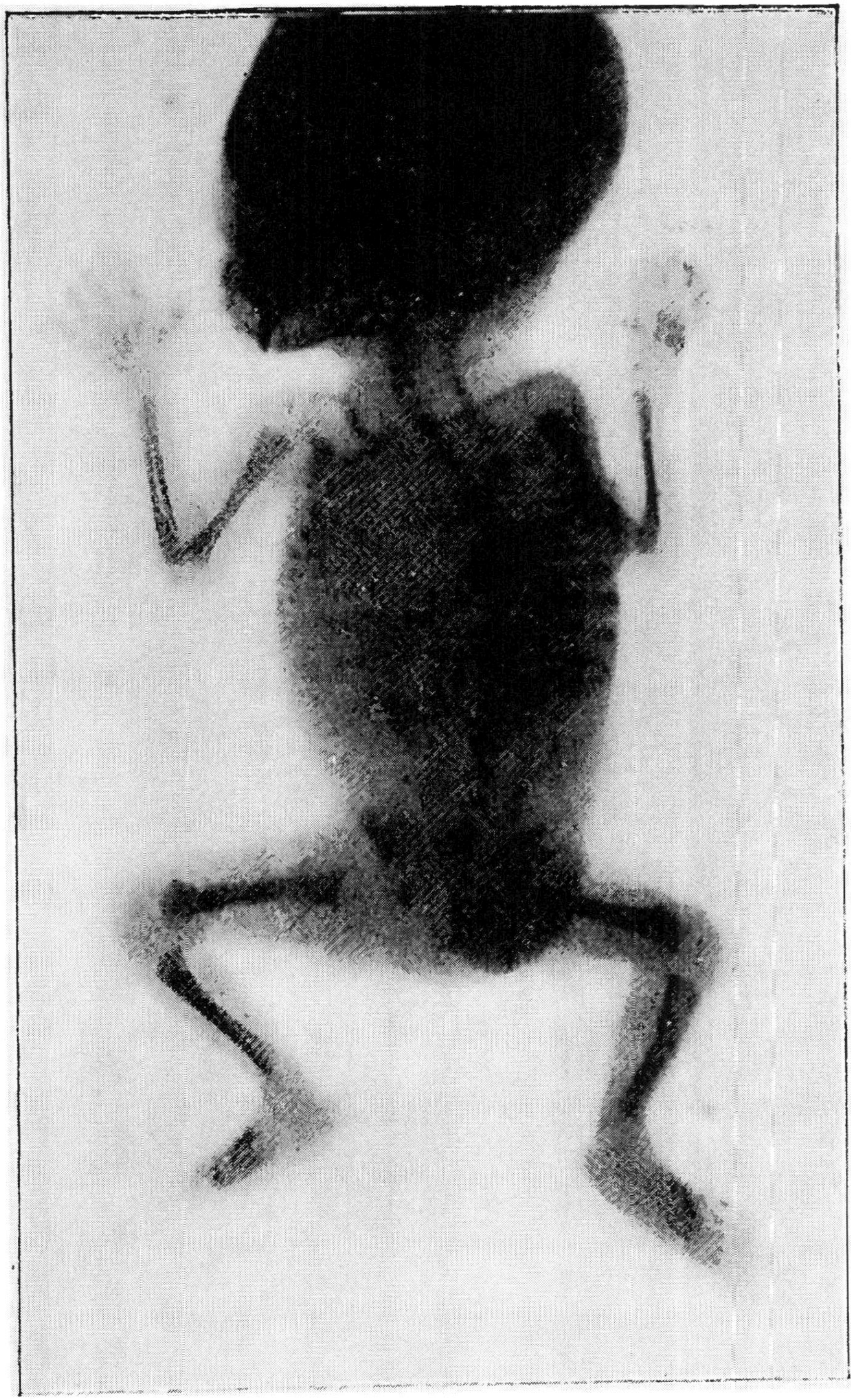

FIG. 45.

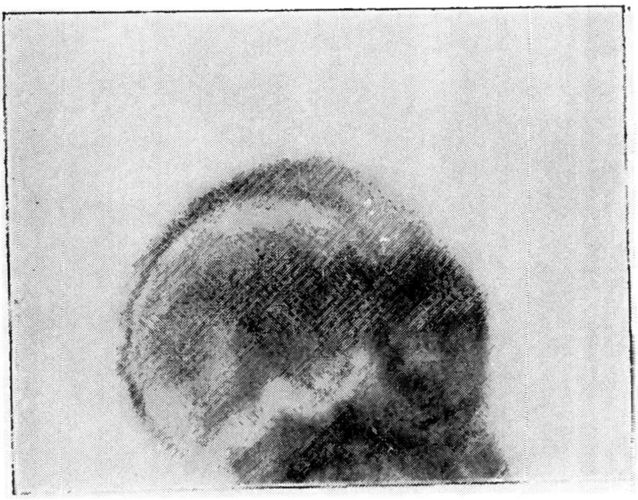

FIG. 46.

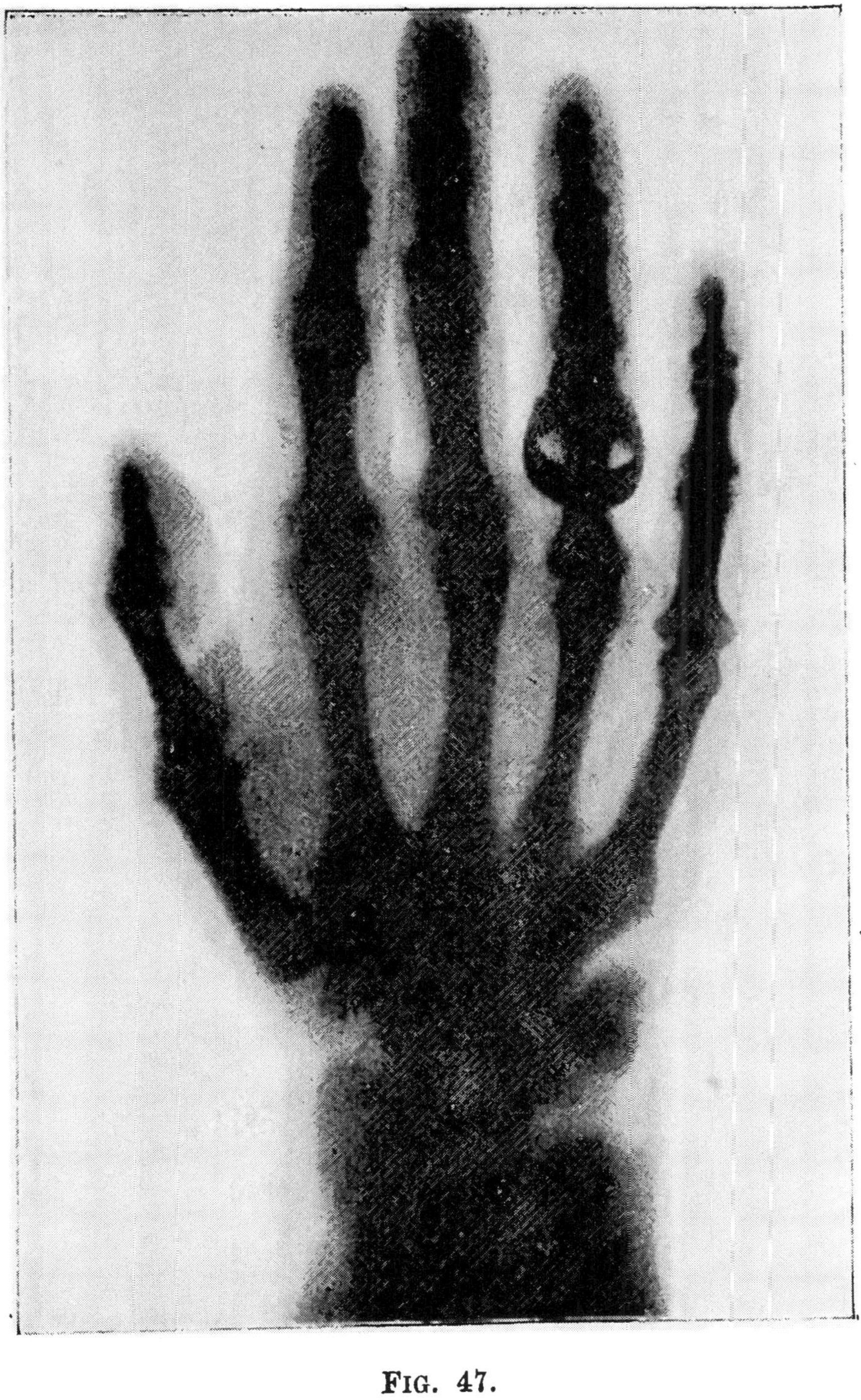

FIG. 47.

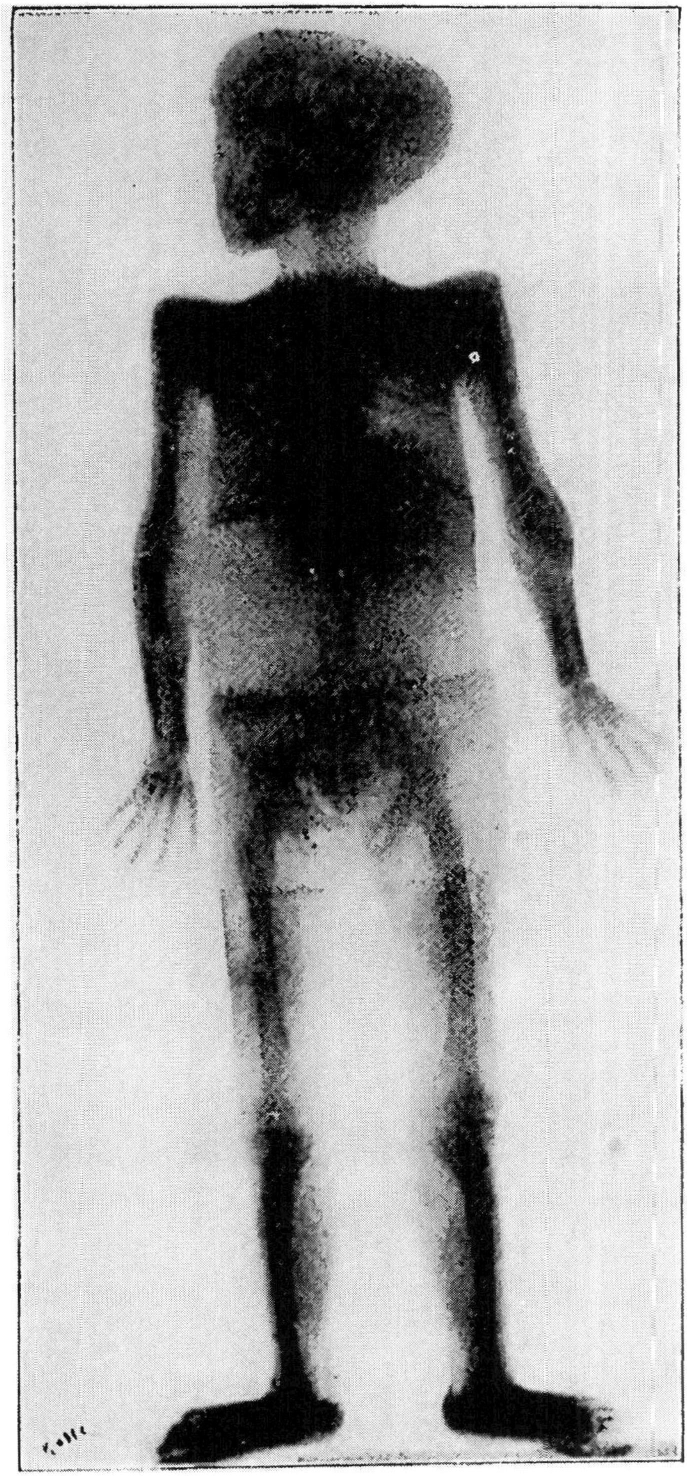

FIG. 48.

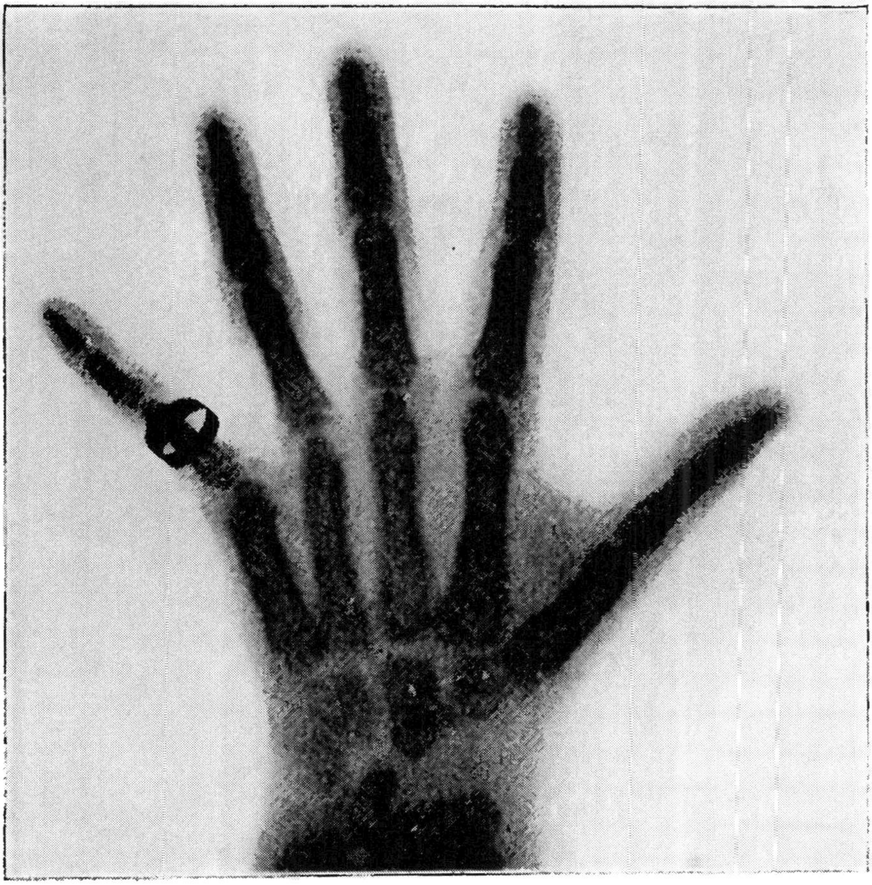

FIG. 49.

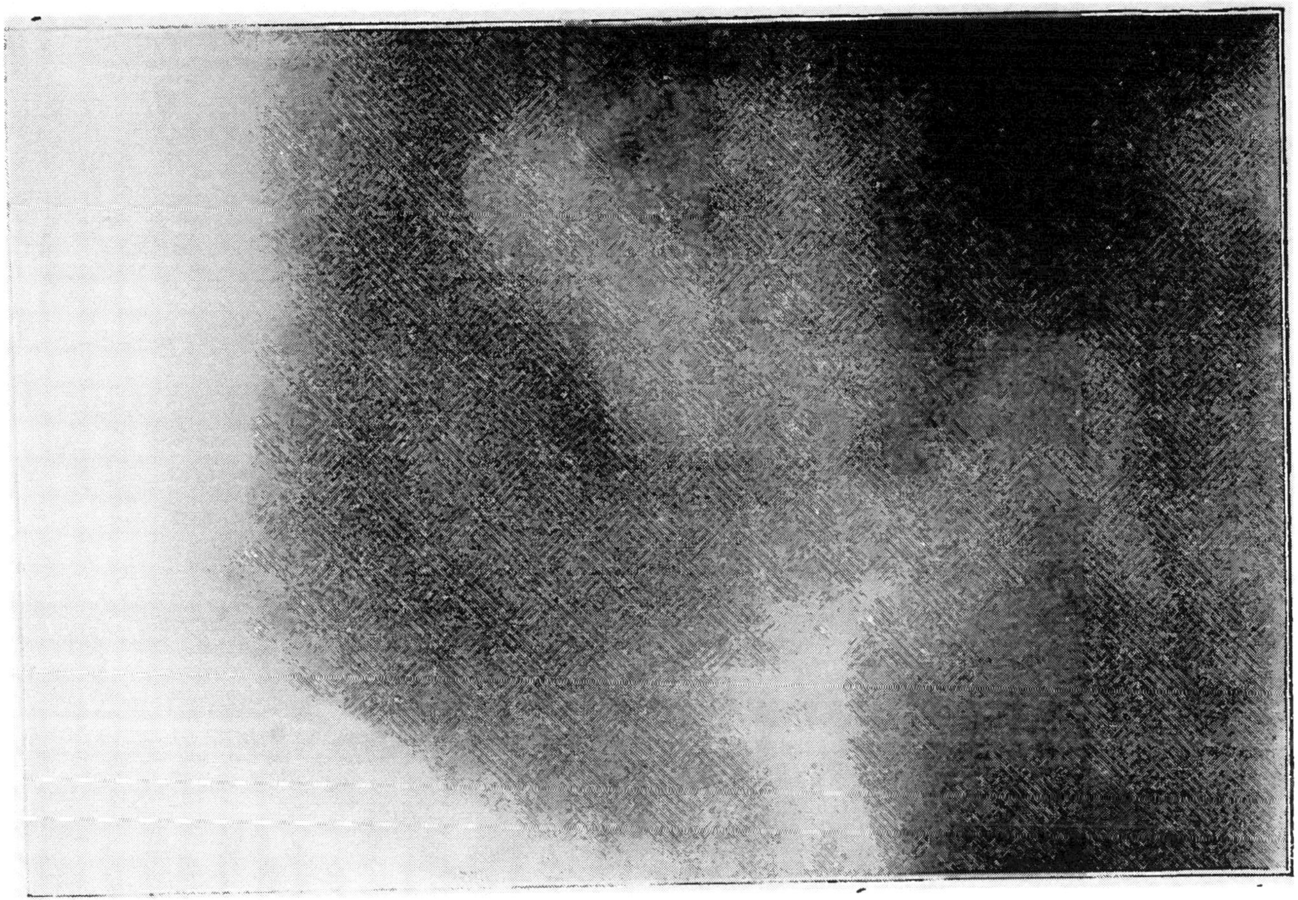

Fig. 50.

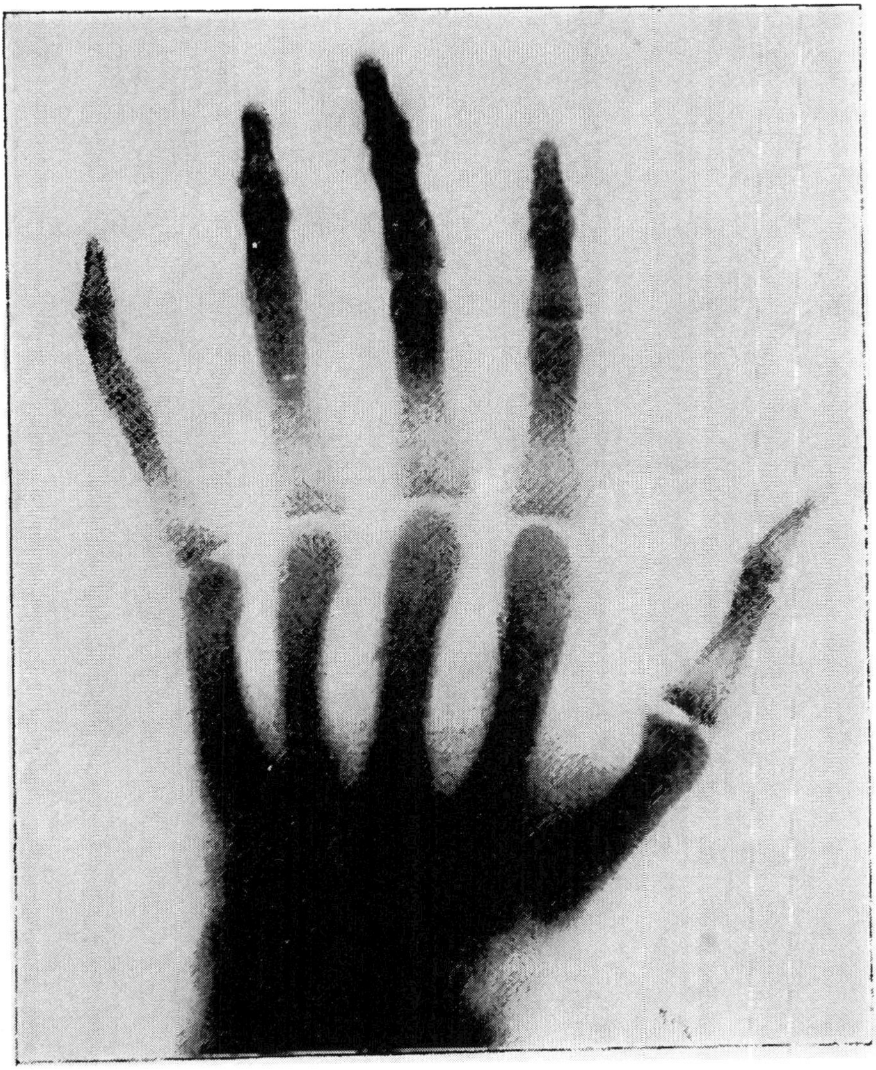

FIG. 51.

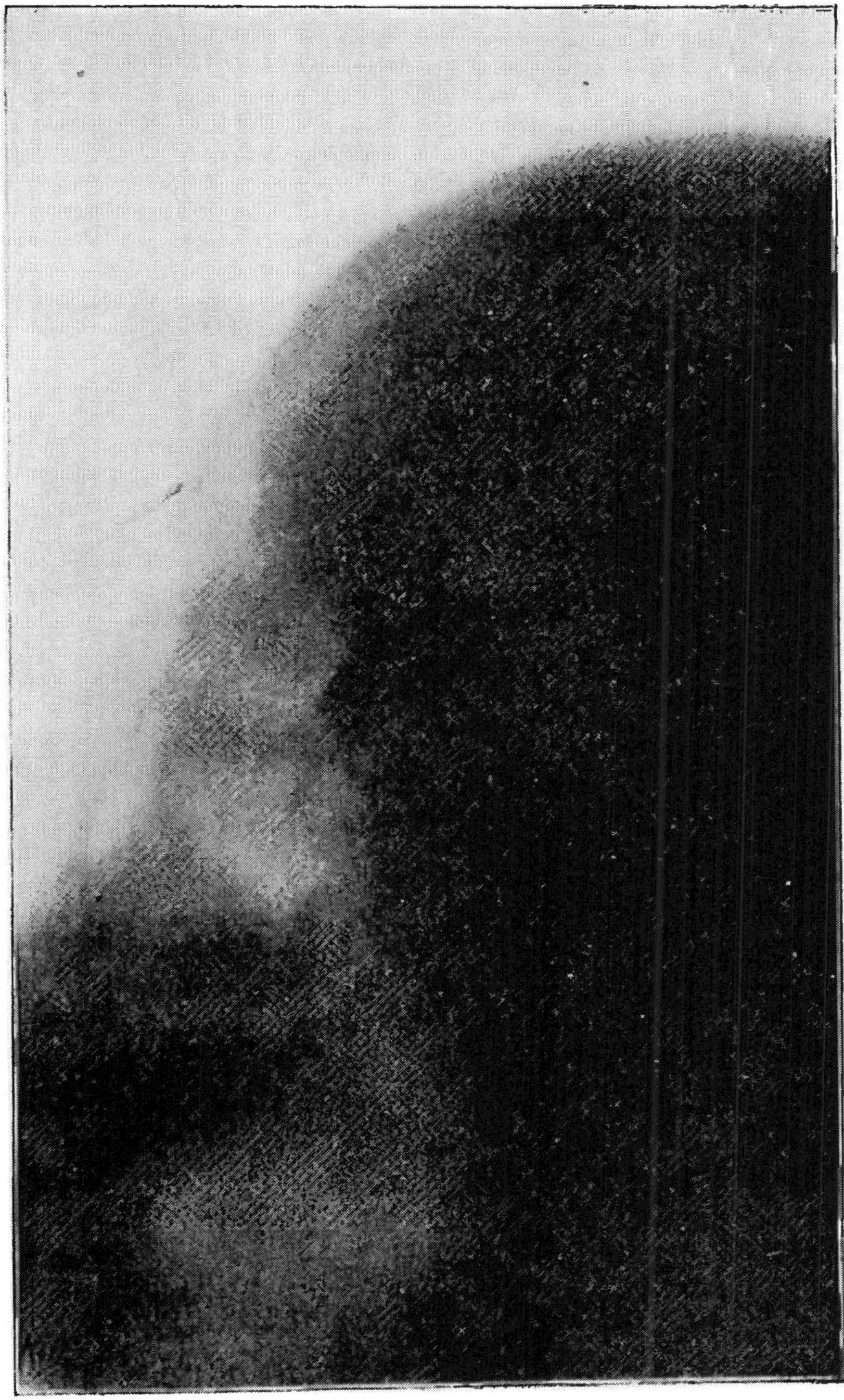

FIG. 52.

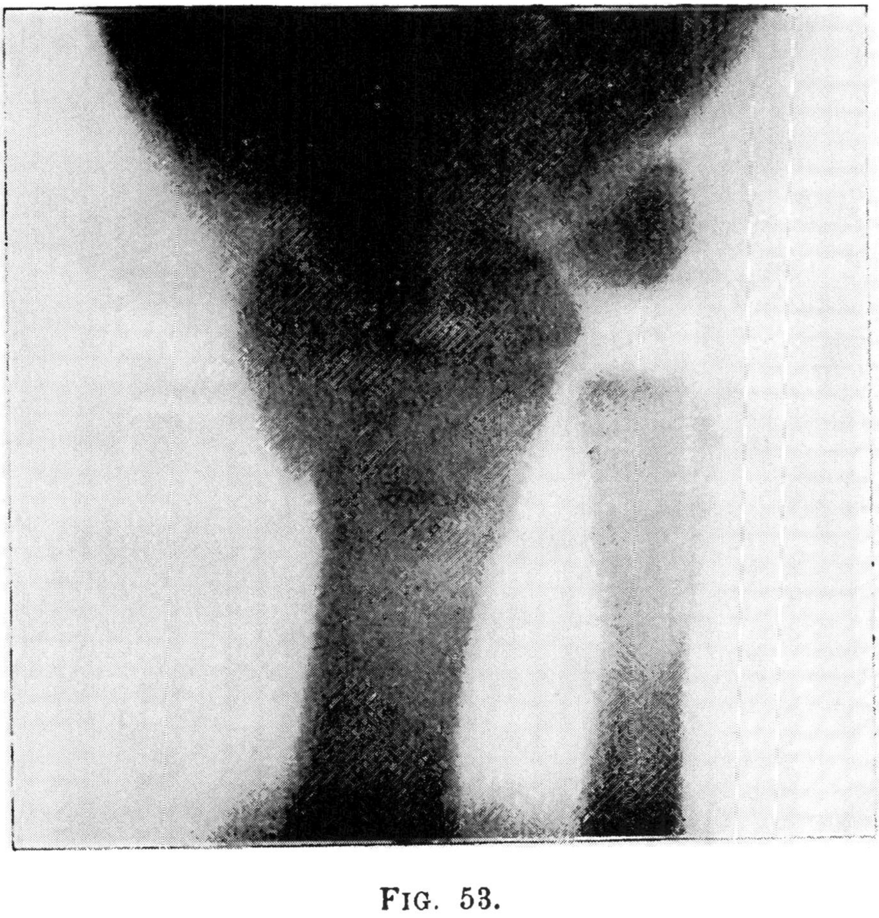

FIG. 53.

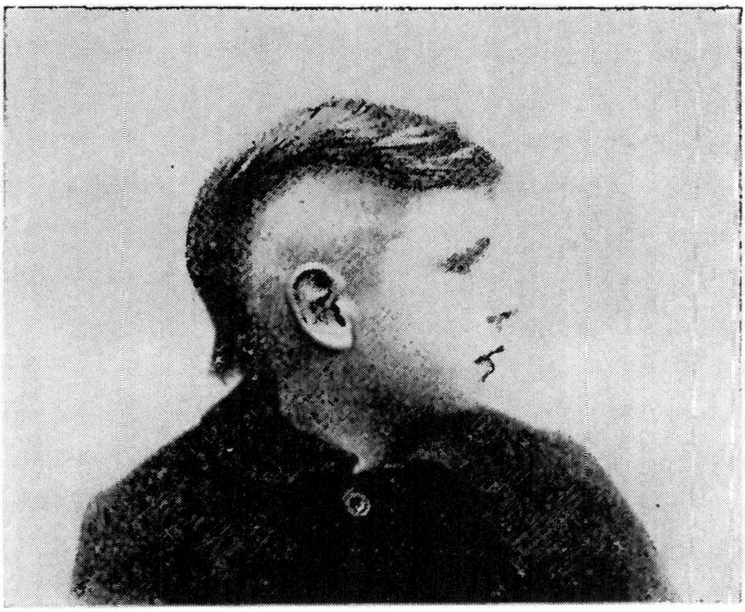

ALOPECIA AREATA,
RESULTING FROM EXPOSURE TO THE X RAYS.

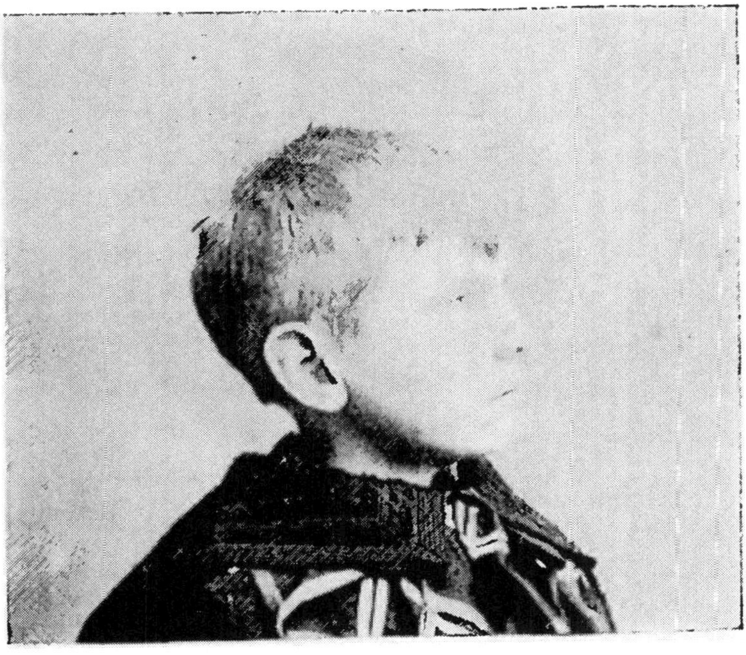

AFTER TREATMENT—HAIR RESTORED.

BI-ELECTROGRAPHS.

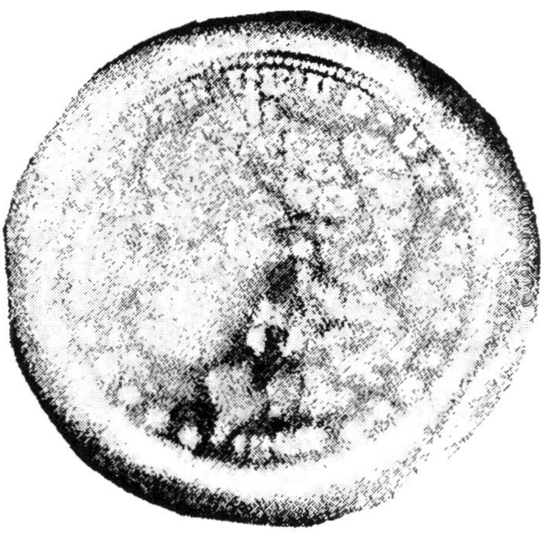

ELECTOGRAPH.

Henry, Niewenglowski and Becquerel that salts of zinc, of calcium, and especially of uranium exposed to strong light, acquire the power of emitting, both then and afterward, an invisible radiation which can penetrate aluminium and act on a photographic plate, has greatly strengthened the position of those philosophers, who maintained that the X rays were of the nature of ultra-violet light, and it has done this in the following way:

"The Becquerel rays are capable of some amount of polarization, and hence are certainly transverse disturbances, like light; they can also be reflected and refracted to a small extent, whereas the X rays can be hardly at all reflected and not at all appreciably refracted. Neither kind can be deflected by a magnet, not even in a vacuum—according to the experiments of M. Lagrange; and an assertion that the X rays could be magnetically deflected after passage through an electrified plate has not been substantiated by careful experiments, made by himself among others. Taking all of these things together, and looking at them in the light of the notable dispersion theory of Von Helmholtz, it has become almost certain that the X rays are simply an extraordinary extension of the spectrum—far beyond the ordinary ultra-violet, and that the Becquerel rays are a less extreme extension in the same direction."

To apply at the present time, the dispersion theory of Helmholtz is by far the most interesting, because it is worked out entirely on the basis of the electro-magnetic theory of light.

"Helmholtz shows, on electro-magnetic principles, that ethereal radiation of smaller and smaller wave lengths should become more and more refrangible, by matter in the molecular form, up to a certain maximum; and this, of course, is ordinary dispersion; but that for waves which are shorter still, the refrangibility, *i.e.*, the refractive index of substances of such very short waves, should rapidly, indeed almost suddenly, drop nearly or quite to zero, thus doubling the spectrum back upon itself, and giving an anomalous dispersion so great that the rays might be bent by a prism in the wrong direction for a certain size of wave. This state of things would be accompanied by extreme opacity, or absorption of the vibrations by the material molecules. If, however, waves existed of a kind still smaller, then the opacity would become less obstrusive; the refractivity would likewise remain very small—either positive or negative perhaps, but probably negative; and ultimately, for extremely small waves of atomic dimensions, the refractivity would become nothing and the opacity very small.

"In a general way it may be said that material atoms act as if they loaded the ether, so that coarse ether waves large enough to affect some dozens or some hundreds of molecules in a row, such as are the waves of visible light, would by reason of this loading be retarded, and therefore both reflected and refracted. All very coarse waves would be refracted about the same amount, but for smaller the period of the waves might synchronize with some of the periods of atomic vibration, such vibration as enables atoms to emit light, and whenever that occurred a violent absorption might be expected, owing to the syntonic response or sympathetic resonance between the matter and the ether. This would have the effect at first of retarding the waves rather more, and of giving the well-known effects of ordinary dispersion, or the sorting out of waves roughly according to size, which we get in the prismatic spectrum. Or if the syntony is strongly marked, fluorescent and phosphorescent effects are to be expected from the jangled atoms; and if for this or any other reason absorption is rapid, the dispersion is what is called "anomalous," which in this connection—indeed in all possible connections—only means unexpectedly complicated.

Push the matter further, however; assume the existence of waves smaller still, so small that they cease to evoke any vibratory response from the material atoms among which they now make their way, the ether of the interstices can hardly be appreciably loaded by the great blocks of immovable substance which now represent the appearance of the atoms, and accordingly retardation and refraction abruptly disappear together, and true absorption also nearly ceases.

"To waves penetrating ethereal interstices, matter, even conducting matter, is fairly transparent; for ordinary notions of conductivity do not apply to those intermolecular spaces; electric displacements no longer excite necessary conduction currents, even in bodies which in the gross are conductors, and accordingly there is little or no dissipation of energy, and any obstruction that exists to the passage of light of this kind is of the ground-glass or turbid-medium type, a certain percentage of the energy being scattered at each obstacle in all directions, instead of being able to excite the material vibrations which we know as heat.

"This is a very bare account of the matter, but it may suffice to indicate the sort of view which is now coming to be almost universally held regarding the nature of those no longer quite X rays. The proof is not complete and will not be till their length has been measured, but in all probability they are ordinary transverse ethereal waves, moving with the customary velocity of light, of various grades of wave length down to $\frac{1}{10^8}$ cm. in length, vibrating therefore some trillions of times in a second (a trillion being 10^{12}), and by the aid of this highest type of X ray we may hope in the future to gain some diffractional insight into the actual structure and appearance of the material molecules among which they go.

"In all probability they are excited by Hertz vibrations

in the atoms themselves. Ordinary light may be due to mechanical or acoustic atomic vibrations; but this X kind of light is more likely due to electric vibrations—*i.e.*, to surgings of the atomic charges. A globe of steel vibrating mechanically might excite either waves a hundred thousand times the sphere in size, if it could excite them at all; but, vibrating electrically, its radiated ethereal waves would be not much bigger than the sphere itself. In other words, its vibration frequency would be multiplied nearly a hundred thousand fold. The mechanical vibration of an atom may emit ordinary light. Its electrical vibration may quite possibly emit X rays."

Becquerel, in an academic paper referred to by Dr. Oliver Lodge, in his summary of the hypothesis of the nature of the rays, shows that these luminiferous rays are emitted by the bisulphate of uranium and potassium and demonstrated their action by photographs made with these invisible rays. He shows that they traverse opaque bodies, particularly aluminium and copper. In a later paper he shows the difference between these rays and the X rays. In considering absorption alone, the two kinds of rays act as though they had different wave lengths, but in the absence of refraction and reflection of the X rays showed a greater difference. Professor Poincare, in his description of the X rays, goes so far as to suggest that all bodies which fluoresce strongly enough may possibly emit X rays in addition to ordinary light, irrespective of how the fluorescence is caused, and that, if the theory be true, X rays need not alone be produced by electrical means, but by any other method.

I have herein tried to show or concentrate the approved and collective theories and beliefs as to the nature of the X rays, and to summarize, we may say that the X rays are transverse ethereal vibrations of extreme short individual wave length and low intensity, and that their activity depends more upon synchronism than upon violence.

KINDRED RESULTS IN ELECTRO-PHOTOGRAPHY.

Early in 1896 I revived electro-photography, and although the results have nothing to do with the Roentgen rays, the experiments are carried on with much the same apparatus as used for radiography, except in the use of the vacuum tube.

The results are both novel and interesting and may be described in a few words. An ordinary photographic plate, wrapped in black paper, is laid upon a small sheet of metal, of about the same size as the dry plate. The latter is connected to the negative pole of the secondary circuit of a small spark coil. (I used the 1 inch.)

The glass side of the plate is turned downward, and a metallic object, preferably a coin, is laid upon the film side of the plate or paper covering same. In the illustration a silver dollar was used. Over the coin another sheet of metal, *i.e.*, aluminium, is laid, which is connected to the positive terminal of the secondary coil. The rheotome is then screwed back as far as possible, or until the primary current refuses to move it; the head of the hammer is then crowded forward, as in flashing, until one or several sparks have passed across the spark gap.

Upon developing the plate a perfect image of the coin will be obtained. Around the periphery of the coin a ring or border of minute sparks may be seen, resembling, or rather indicating, the minute subdivisions of the spark or sparks allowed to have passed in the experiment.

By closely examining the experiment, a pale blue or violet-colored light will be found to encircle the coin as the sparks are allowed to pass.

BI-ELECTROGRAPHS.[66]

While experimenting in the production of the electro-

66 Physikalishe Bericht, Freie Presse, Feb. 22, 1896.

graph, I conceived the idea of manifolding the picture produced, by using two dry plates in place of the one in the former experiment. (Feb. 21, 1896.) In the experiment, the upper side of the coin, covered in the former experiment with the metal plate, was in this case covered with the film side of a second dry plate, upon the glass side of which a metal plate was placed, connected and exposed as in the former experiment. The blue or violet-colored light was again observed.

Upon developing the two plates, both sides of the coin were shown beautifully, with the same periphery of minute sparks. To obtain the best results the plates are used bare and the experiment is carried on in a dark room, by ruby light.

MAGNETOGRAPHS.

An interesting production is the magnetograph. The experiment as conducted by Professor McKay[67] is as follows:

The ordinary dry plate wrapped in light-proof paper is again used, with the metallic object to be pictured laid upon the film side of the plate. The two may be wrapped together to prevent moving or shifting of the coin or metal. A piece of cardboard is then laid upon the pole terminals of a powerful horseshoe or electromagnet, and the plate with its object to be magnetographed, facing the cardboard, is laid upon the latter. The armature is then gently presented to the glass side of the plate, and allowed to remain as attracted by the magnet for a few minutes (5 to 10). If an electro-magnet or the magnetic field of a dynamo is used, a piece of soft iron can be employed in place of the armature. The plate is developed after the proper time of exposure, and the negative obtained will show a shadow

67 Prof. McKay: Scientific American, April 18, 1896; E. B. Frost: Elect. Eng., March 11, 1896.

of the metallic object employed in the experiment. The result, however, is due to magnetism and not to X rays.

THERMOGRAPHS.

Another interesting experiment is the production of the thermograph—a picture produced by heat effects. The experiment may be carried on as follows[68]—although a number of failures must at first be expected:

A sensitized gelatino-bromide of silver dry plate is placed, film side up, into a tray and covered with clean, cold water and allowed to remain in this for a moment or two, or until the gelatin film of the plate becomes slightly softened. The water is then poured off, and a coin or other piece of metal, which has previously been heated in hot water for a short time, or rendered cold by laying upon a piece of ice for two or three minutes, is laid gently down upon the film. With a gentle though firm pressure it is forced into place. At this moment most failures result. The pressure is either too severe or not severe enough, and the film, which has been softened by the water, is forced upward and lacerated, spoiling the effect. I have found that by using a coin with a worn edge better results are obtained, with less danger of lacerating the film. Copper coins should be used, as silver will not give the effect. The developer is then poured into the tray with the coin still in its position and well covered with developer, allowed to remain for several minutes, and is then removed gently, leaving the developer in the tray, until the plate is developed or the details of the image of the coin are definitely defined. If the coin has been allowed to remain too long before removal, no result may be produced. In pressing the coin firmly into place the

---

68 C. F. Townsend: "Thermographic Images," Photogram, London, April 18, 1896.

air retained between the depressions in the figures of the coin is difficult to exclude, but after several attempts the necessary pressure may be ascertained. In removing the coin from the film the suction occasioned between the two holds the former down with considerable force and care must be taken in removing it. A peculiarity, which is at first very striking, is the long time necessary to develop the plate, varying from 10 to 16 minutes or more, before anything will appear upon the plate. With patience, however, a good negative is eventually obtained. To develop in half an hour, with new developer, is considered good time; but as much as an hour may be necessary. The tray may be covered and allowed to stand, with an occasional inspection of the plate from time to time, to determine its progress. The negative is fixed in the usual hypo-bath, washed and dried as any other negative.

CHAPTER IX.

THE PRACTICAL APPLICATION AND USES OF THE X RAYS IN SURGERY, MEDICINE, DENTISTRY, ETC.

THE most important factor in favor of the Roentgen discovery is its direct use and application in surgery.

The discoverer himself made the first anatomical radiograph by exposing his own hand to the rays on a sensitized plate, which upon developing was found to exhibit the same relation of flesh and bone as had been shown upon the fluorescent screen when viewed by that instrument.

Millions of objects have undoubtedly been pictured, by this time, of all kinds and of innumerable descriptions; but to the medical profession the X rays have proved themselves of sufficient value and distinction to have the discovery now, and forever, placed in rank with the discovery of the ligature, anæsthesia, antiseptics, etc.

The name of Roentgen will be hereafter inscribed forever upon the histories of evolution and equally ranked with Hunter, Lister, Koch, etc., of the nineteenth century.

The use of the X rays may be classified as follows:[69]

1. To study normal anatomy.
2. To observe the relation of fragments in fractures of bone.

---

69 See also eight divisions under the "Methods of Diagnosing," Amer. Journal of Med. Sciences, Aug., 1896; Dr. M. J. Stern, "Diagnostic Value of X Rays," Phil. County Med. Society, Nov. 11, 1896.

3. To study and diagnose dislocations.

4. To study and diagnose diseased bone.

5. To diagnose anchylosis of joints.

6. To locate foreign bodies, *i.e.*, bullets, needles, glass, wood, etc., in flesh or bone.

7. It is of diagnostic value in cases of tumors or enlargements of inner organs, such as the spleen, liver, kidneys, heart, etc.

8. In obstetrics, radiograms may be used to show the exact relation between the bony pelvis and the fœtus in utero.

To further aquaint the reader with the individual and tabulated uses of these rays, I will describe each division in the table just given, in a concise and explicit manner, with the view of assisting the beginner in producing radiograms or radiographs of such description as may be included therein.

1. In Normal Anatomy. Not only can we study the outline of the living bone and its relation to its articulant, but we can also observe its growth from infancy on.

The study of embryology is therefore especially rendered interesting by the use of radiographs, and is of great service to the physiologist in demonstrating the growth of bone and the bone centers of almost every bone in the body.

The comparative size of the head and body of the fœtus is beautifully shown. Also the size and relation of the cerebrum and cerebellum, which can readily be radiographed, owing to the thin bony walls of the skull.

The absence of certain bones at certain ages of the fœtus is shown in Fig. 45, in which is depicted a radiograph of a fœtus. Especial notice is drawn to the following perfect portrayal of the cerebrum and cerebellum of a fœtus at the above age. (Fig. 46.)

In the next figure the reader will find a radiogram of the

normal adult hand, showing the relation of the entire wrist joint, radius and ulna. The sesamoid bones of the thumb are also shown in the illustration. (Fig. 47.)

Fig. 48 represents a picture of the entire body, made and completed by me, October 24, 1896.[70] The body is necessarily made in sections, as dry plates of the required size could not be readily obtained, unless made to order, and would be very awkward to handle. The sections appear as variously shaded portions. In the negative the heart, liver, stomach, spleen, and kidneys can readily be distinguished. They are obliterated to a certain extent in the half-tone reproduction. I believe this to be the first entire adult body radiographed in America.

Fig. 49 shows a picture of the normal hand of a boy 10 years of age. I beg to call the attention of the reader to the several differences as compared with the adult hand —*i.e.*, the absence of certain bones in the carpal region and also the epiphesial separations of the bone ends.

Illustration No. 45 is only of interest in reference to its historical relation to the subject, and herein I beg to present a reproduction of a radiogram of the first entire human body made in the world (February 14, 1896). It was exhibited by me at a lecture shortly thereafter.[71] I believe Professor Puluj, of Prague, made the second radiogram of similar nature early in March, 1896.

The student of comparative anatomy has found an aid in the X rays. By radiographs he is enabled to record the bony structure and growth of the bones of animals of all description, and to compare them with those of the human body.

The relation of the blood vessels to the bones can also be shown by injecting the vessels with some opaque solu-

---

70 Kolle: Nov. Trans. Brooklyn Surgical Society, Brocklyn Medical Journal, January, 1897.

71 Kolle: Lecture to Physicians, Brooklyn, April 23, 1896.

tion—*i.e.*, Teichmann's mixture of lime, cinnabar and petroleum. In truth, dissection of the cadaver may in this way be rendered more instructive and interesting.

2. Dislocations may not only be recognized to a certainty, but a radiograph of such, made in but a few moments, can be recorded for future reference. The dislocated member could also be viewed with the fluoroscope, or a negative made, before the reduction of the deformity, with hardly any loss of time or added suffering to the patient.

Fig. 50 shows a rare form of dislocation. The head of a diseased femur is found to be dislocated forward and upward, and can be compared with its normal fellow on the opposite side.

3. Diseased bone is especially well shown in radiographs, such as tubercular bone lesion, etc. Osteoma or enlarged bone may be included under this same division.

4. Anchylosis may be determined, whether ligamentous or bony, so determining its curability or *vice versa*, guiding the surgeon in determining the latter, and in the event of a necessary operation aids in making the prognosis in prophesying, by the aid of the negative, the probability of a more useful joint, after operation.

5. To locate foreign bodies the X rays are of inestimable value. Very early pictures were made of pieces of glass, wood, needles, etc., in the hands and limbs of patients, locating the foreign body exactly, with but a few minutes' exposure, whereas probing, successful or otherwise, might have caused hours of painful suffering.

In Fig. 51 I beg to show a radiograph of the hand of a young man, aged 17 years, who had been stabbed in the hand with a lead-pencil, some time ago. An operation was performed shortly thereafter, and several pieces of lead and wood were removed; but the pain in the hand, which soon began to swell after the healing of the wound made at the time of the operation, became severe and a second operation was performed and several pieces of lead and wood were again removed. The wound was necessarily made large to enable the surgeon to fully explore it for the foreign body. No more could be found. The wound healed as before and the patient was again discharged, with but the same unpleasant symptoms returning shortly thereafter. The radiogram shows a sliver of wood of extreme small size lying alongside of the middle metacarpal bone at about the center of the hand. The radiogram was made in the afternoon, at the suggestion of Dr. W. C. W., and the patient was operated on by him the same evening. The piece of wood was readily found and removed, without any returning trouble.

The illustration Fig. 52 shows the skull of E. T., aged 19, a student. He was admitted to the Methodist Episcopal Hospital, September 14, 1896, with the following history: Two days prior to admission he shot himself, with suicidal intent, in the right temple. He said that he did not lose consciousness following the infliction of the injury, but immediately became totally blind. Examination showed a bullet wound about an inch behind the external angular process of the right frontal bone and somewhat below the level of the eyebrow. There was marked tenderness throughout the supraorbital region, and some headache complained of. Although it was evident that the bullet had not penetrated the cranial cavity, but on the contrary had transversed both orbits.[72] At the request of Dr. G. R. Fowler, I made a radiogram of the head and located the ball, as shown in the illustration. The ball was removed October 17, 1896, and the patient was discharged from the hospital shortly thereafter, well in body, though blind in both eyes.

---

72 Fowler: Trans. Brooklyn Surgical Society, November, 1896; Brooklyn Medical Journal, December 10, 1896.

This is believed to be the pioneer case of location of a bullet in the head by means of the Roentgen rays, in which an operation was undertaken and successfully carried out upon the basis of the findings of an X ray picture.

Suffice to say that foreign bodies of whatever nature may be located by the negative or fluoroscope in a few moments, so facilitating the removal of the same.

In making radiographs of surgical nature, I beg to call the attention of the reader to the fact that certain chemical compounds are opaque to the rays, and in the negative may be mistaken for foreign bodies contained within the limb of the patient. This is especially true of iodoform, which is greatly used in the dressing of wounds. It is exceedingly opaque and casts a shadow on the negative which might be readily mistaken for fragments of a bullet, etc., and so mislead the surgeon in operating, causing unnecessary cutting, loss of blood, and possibly a larger wound to heal, as well as puzzling the operator.

Iodine and sulphur are also opaque.[73].

6. In the diagnosis of fractures the rays are extremely useful; not only can we view the fragments of the shattered bone, at the same time being enabled to reduce the fracture, but we can avoid the danger of abnormal coaptation of the fractured ends of the bone and study the mending joints from time to time, observing the amount of callus drawn out, or the ligamentous union in other similar cases. The swollen joint, where the œdema follows the injury, is no longer misleading—if a fracture is present, anæsthesia is not necessary to determine it. The patient is merely brought near the active tube and the injured member is quickly and accurately examined with the fluoroscope. Not only can we see the bones at once by the use of the screen, but we can record the fracture or injury,

---

73 M, Meslaus: Comptes Rendus; Scientific American, March 28, 1896.

use it historically or legally, in the place of the heretofore expensive expert testimony. My true belief of such a radiograph, made by a responsible operator, in the presence of the plaintiff's and defendant's counselors and medical advisers, is, and should be, recognized and accepted as exact and conclusive evidence. The negative so procured could not deceive even a layman, much less an educated and exacting juryman, if both normal and abnormal or injured parts were pictured to him. The only objection that could be found with this method is the damaging evidence brought against the defendant; but in the face of responsibility this reliable evidence should not be tampered with, and admitted "*pro bono publico.*"

Colle's fracture is often met with in the practice of medicine, and in Fig. 53 we have such a fracture depicted in a most interesting and educational manner. Not only are the radius and ulna fractured, but the reader may readily observe a fracture of the styloid process of the radius and ulna—a condition very seldom met with or diagnosed. There is also a dislocation of the wrist joint.

7. Tumors and the enlargement of organs can readily be diagnosed. By the use of either screen or photographic plate, pathological enlargements of the liver, sarcoma, etc., syphilitic gummatas situated in any part of the body, enlarged spleen of whatever cause, floating kidney, etc., can all be examined by either method, and permanently recorded by radiographs made of the patient.

Tumors of the brain, hemorrhagic or specific, etc., offer an interesting study. They can be localized if of fair dimension, as the living heart.

In Germany and England tubercular growth and individual tubercles in the lungs are diagnosed by this method of using the fluoroscope.

Stones in the bladder or kidneys are quickly shown, as well as stones in the gall bladder, independent of their specific formation. A number of these radiograms have been recorded here in this country and abroad.[74]

The human heart can not only be seen by the use of the screen, but its movements could be radiographed by flashing, as already described, or by combining the fluoroscope and kinetoscope, in the form of the fluoro-kinetoscope—an instrument made for making photo-fluorographs of any moving body. The movable film of the kinetoscope, made to revolve very quickly, photographs the fluorograph or skiagraph, thrown upon the screen by the flashing method used in connection with tube and coil.

Atheroma, a calcareous condition of the blood vessels, can be diagnosed and readily seen.

Excellent radiographs of the heart are exhibited by many experimenters, but they are as yet rather vague in outline, owing to the fact that that organ is composed of soft tissue and is in constant motion; however, from a radiograph made as suggested by Dr. McIntyre, namely, by flashing, a good result should be expected. The heart is easily seen, by the use of the screen and a focus tube, charged with a powerful spark coil of at least 10 inches spark capacity.[75]

8. In obstetrics the radiogram promises to be of considerable value, both in determining the position of the fœtus and deformity of the pelvis; also demonstrating the relation between the former and the bony pelvis.

In fact any part of the body can be examined or radiographed and recorded, that is, within the limits of the practicability of the X rays. Statistics of all operative cases

---

74 A. P. Laurie and J. T. Leon: "The X Rays in the Detection of Renal and Vesical Calculi," London Lancet, Jan. 16, 1897; American Medico Surgical Bulletin, May, 1897.

75 Benedict: "The Normal Heart may be seen to Rise Above the Diaphragm, and that the Space between them is Visible to the eye," Wiener: Med. Blatter, Oct. 29, 1896.

relative to bone or the removal of foreign bodies should be accompanied by an X ray picture.

Deformities are shown to exist in their natural pathological condition, which is in itself a great help to the surgeon in outlining the steps of an operation and in deciding as to the necessity of an operation. The strengthened prognosis in these cases, and its value to the operator, should not be overlooked. Probing, which has always reminded me of arctic exploration, may be laid aside with gratifying comfort both to doctor and patient. There need be no waste of time in determining the exact location of a bullet or what-not. The foreign missile is located and can be quickly removed. Only those surgeons who have probed such wounds, perhaps unsuccessfully, for minutes and perhaps many of them, will readily appreciate the value of the discovery of Roentgen.

In time of war a portable apparatus would be a decidedly humane addition to the surgeon's armament.

The portable apparatus for this purpose could be of condensed form. Where storage cells could not be obtained, primary batteries could be used, made from rubber cells, which can be of the telescopic variety, requiring little space and being light for transportation. The chemicals for the batteries could be carried in the usual medicine chest. The setting up of such an apparatus should not require more than half an hour at the longest.

Every ship of war, army and navy hospital should have one—not alone for the benefit of the surgeon, but likewise for the poor, miserable, and suffering patient. The prompt attention necessarily associated with the rapidity of an exposure guarantees the patient a better chance of recovery.

All the larger hospitals in the United States are already provided with an apparatus, and the radiographers of these institutions are working faithfully and with gratifying results. The apparatus need be of little expense if properly managed. The initial outlay for such should be amply repaid by two or three radiograms.

I would certainly encourage colleges, both academic and medical, in instituting this discovery and its uses as a study; also practical demonstrations of the use and nature of the X rays to students, with the purpose of advancing the art, and applicable particularly to surgery, etc.

It is claimed by Dr. T. S. Middleton, of New York—who believes in the theory of Tesla—that the rays are streams of particles, and that these moving or bombarding particles or atoms could be made to convey medicinal agents into such parts of the body as are diseased, so bringing about a cure. He believes it to be applicable to the consumptive or tubercular patient, and that a cure might be brought about in this way.

Little has been done in this direction, although I have several reports of recoveries from this disease, where it was located in the joints. All are given by German physicians; but as yet I have been unable to substantiate them as correct and reliable. That such a curative power may be held by this peculiar ray is not at all impossible, and much may be expected from them in the future. The patients suffering from pulmonary tuberculosis were exposed from 10 to 40 minutes at a time, for several sittings a week, to an active focus tube. In tuberculosis of the joints it has been found that the discharge from the same became thin, viscid and of exceedingly bad odor—instead of the usual ropy nature, and that by continued treatment the swelling gradually receded, with lessening discharge, eventually disappearing. It has been claimed by a German authority that by a continued treatment with the X rays for three or four weeks a cure may be brought about. No such results have been recorded in this country that I am aware of.

That the rays are of germicidal value has been disputed

by several American authorities. Two prominent physicians of Chicago[70] claim that the rays possess a killing power, and yet again several and equally eminent men,[71] contradict this, and do not accredit the rays with any such gracious propensities. I believe that the work in this direction should be progressive and not a mere spasmodic experiment.

Personally I have found no change in the exposed bacteria—instead of a germicidal action the rays seemed to aid the growth and increase the number of spores. I used aluminium tubes and a gelatin culture basis.

I may say that certain germs thrived, under exposure, more than others. It is true that ultra-violet light has a destructive effect upon bacteria.[72] And owing to the fact that the X rays simulate the ultra-ultra-violet rays, a germicidal property may be yet found in the former.[73]

The fleshy structures are as yet to be differentiated. In underexposures, faint lines corresponding to the muscles may be observed; but definite results are not shown. The fact that the inner organs can be obtained on negatives is in itself of great interest and importance. That the human and living heart can be pictured by this method of radiography is alone a progressive step, and helps to unfathom the abyss of mystery connected with the discovery.

---

70 Profs. W. P. Pratt and H. Wightmann claim by experiments made upon cultures of the bacilli of diphtheria, influenza, cholera, tuberculosis, anthrax, etc., that the X rays acted fatally upon same. Electricity, New York, April 22, 1896.

71 Bleyer, Electricity, April 22, 1896: "Our paraphernalia of to-day is not sufficient to lay claim to the extraordinary discovery made by Drs. Pratt and Wightmann."

72 T. G. Lyons, London Medical Record, March 7, 1896, states that diphtheria germs exposed 12 hours to the rays showed no signs of modification in growth.

73 See experiments of Vortet: Electrical Review, April 28, 1897, reprinted from London Lancet.

The vigor with which thousands of experimenters took up the discovery is certainly an indication of a bright future. Since the day that Roentgen first saw the rays and applied them to use, hundreds of valuable data have been added—thousands of flames have been kindled in the hearts and minds of scientists, with an eager desire of adding to the list of discoveries. Perhaps millions have hoped in their further use and application.

As early as February, 1896, I believed in the possibility of using the rays with the idea of viewing the human heart, and was at that time criticised for this belief. To see that organ is now a thing of the past. What will the future bring?

Since the time mentioned new and powerful tubes, new screens and currents of great efficiency have been added to the improvements of that time, and still the end is not yet here!

The rays have even been suggested in the treatment of blindness,[74] but by careful and patient experiments made in my laboratory, I have been led to discredit that power. Owing to the nature of the rays such results as have been reported could not have been obtained. The lenses of the eye are to a great extent impervious to these rays, their opacity is equal to that of a plate of glass 1 mm. thick,[75] and even if a certain part of this radial stream is allowed to fall upon the retina, optic nerve, or the center of this special sense, no refraction, reflection or concentration of the rays is possible—therefore the object held in the stream of rays could not be focused upon such retina, optic nerve or center, and consequently the image, unless exceedingly

74 "The X Ray in Blindness," New York Medical Journal, July 4, 1896; Dorn & Brandes: "Das Auge und die Roentgen Strahlen," Wiedemann's Annalen, vol. lx.

75 "The lenses of the eye are equal to the opacity of a plate of glass 1 mm. thick," Prof. Salvini, Scientific American, March 28, 1896.

small, would appear only as a shadow of the whole object, obliterating the sensation of light—in these cases amounting to a peculiar twinkling—like a number of dancing stars, which I have termed *Stern-shuppenlicht.* I have used the radioscope[76] in these experiments, which I made by substituting the screen end of the fluoroscope with a sheet of aluminium, so that by holding the scope to the eyes no light, except that due to the direct action of the rays upon the eyes, could be seen. I may say here that most of the experiments made in this direction were made with the fluoroscope, or the patient was brought near the uncovered active tube, and that the results recorded are to a great extent, if not all, due to ordinary light and not to the action of the rays. Dorn and Brandes claim that the lenses of the eye absorb the rays, and for that reason the eye cannot appreciate them.[77]

Dr. Brandes claims that patients, having the lenses of their eyes removed, were enabled to see the rays. If these patients were blind I doubt his report, for divers reasons and those given above. The seeing power of any eye depends upon the condition of the retina of such, and if that were destroyed no other effects than those already mentioned could be expected.

Closely associated with the subject of general surgery is that of dentistry.[78] The teeth being more compact than bone naturally offer more resistance to the passage of the rays than bone would, or in other words the teeth are of

---

76 Koile: "Effect of X Rays on Vision," New York Medical Journal, January 16, 1897.

77 Wiedemann's Annalen, vol. lx.

78 H. I. Dreshfield, Manchester, succeeded in showing the first set of teeth in place and the second set still *in situ*, in the bone back of and above the others in a boy 13 years of age. Scientific American, April 11, 1896; C. E. Kells, Jr., American X-Ray Journal, August, 1897, "Radiography in Dentistry."

greater density than bone. A radiogram of a jaw-bone containing teeth is at once an interesting one. The bone is represented in lighter shade than the teeth, and each tooth, with its root or fangs projecting into the bone, is shown in darker shade. Metal fillings in a tooth would show exceedingly well.

Another important fact is that the central canal of the tooth, containing the blood vessels and nerve for the nourishment of the tooth, can also be seen, but of course in lighter shade than either bone or tooth. The teeth of children, still retained and hidden within the gums, can be shown.

Pus, being opaque to a certain extent, could be located by this method of diagnosis, and in such a way disease of and about the tooth can be shown. Pieces of bone, fracture of the maxillary bones resulting from any cause, and even an old root buried and hidden in obscurity within the gum, could be observed. A broken drill or other metal instrument could be found at once.

For examining the teeth and the alveolar structure, where radiography is not employed, I have devised a special form of fluoroscope—the Dentaskiascope, by which the operator is enabled to inspect teeth and their roots, one by one, with ease and comfort to both operator and patient. The instrument is simply a potassium-platino-cyanide or fluorescent screen, held or retained within an aluminium case, in such a position that its skiagraph is thrown backward upon an inclined mirror, placed at a proper plane with the former, so that the operator is enabled to view the reflected image on the screen through a black tube, adjustable at either end or at the top of the case. The two openings not used are closed with screw caps while the one to which the tube is attached is being used. The instrument is otherwise used as the ordinary fluoroscope.

For making radiograms of the teeth the movable screen

end of the above is removed and replaced with a light-proof covered sensitized film or dry plate. This is exposed as ordinarily to a momentary exposure, which is all that is required to obtain a good negative of tooth and root.

The plate-holder should be placed down far enough to include the entire tooth from the crown to the extremity of the root. The soft tissue at the floor of the mouth will permit this, but for teeth in the upper maxillary the plate in its holder must be placed on a slant to obtain a good negative. A small clamp of wood may be employed to retain the plate-holder in the required position, but this is hardly necessary, as the time of exposure is but of very short duration.

CHAPTER X.

THE EFFECT OF THE X RAYS UPON LIVING TISSUES.

WELL may Nicola Tesla term electricity a charming and enchanting study, and truly may he be priviliged to use such terms, as every one who has been fortunate enough to listen to one of his lectures,[79] which were highly praised and repeated here and abroad in several countries—upon his experiments and inventions in the so-called high-frequency and high-potential alternating currents. His exhibitions in connection with that subject were not alone original, striking, and novel, but marvelous and most unnatural. And even his modest descriptions of his attainments and those of scientific predecessors can hardly cause the minds of the general community to realize that there is a great gulf of reality between him and the wonderful Aladdin and his lamp.

Tesla and his lamp interests and awes us. So is it with the Roentgen discovery. Roentgen and his lamp interests, pleases, and awes us, and still, in the active, greenish-hued vacuum tube can we see aught to displease the mind.

The disappointment of the layman in first viewing the tube in action is considerable. He evidently expects to behold a large and wonderfully brilliant light, that makes all around him appear ghostly and penetrable, and his companions to look like living skeletons, clanging their naked bones together at every move; but the unexpected

79 "Inventions, Researches and Writings of Tesla," T. C. Martin.

color of the tube arouses him from his momentary disappointment.

The tube surely seems harmless, much more so than the brushes and tubes of Tesla. But the invisible force shooting out from it has led us to regard the tube with more respect than carelessness, and I will briefly rehearse some of the effects of the rays upon tissues exposed to them.[80]

When the hand or any part of the body is subjected to the rays for a considerable length of time and at frequent intervals, a reddened and inflamed condition of the skin results, not unlike sunburn. A dermatitis,[81] as Dr. M. J. Stern[82] calls it, or an erythema.[83] This condition proves to be very stubborn indeed under treatment, and active remedial agents applied for weeks only reduce the trouble. I have seen four of these cases, one of which was exceedingly severe. The patient was accustomed to handling the fluoroscope almost constantly during the day. After several weeks of this exposure his right hand began to redden and swell, until it was thought advisable to have the hand amputated if the trouble continued. Active treatment for over five weeks has been continued and the patient seems to be recovering slowly now.

Another peculiar effect of the ray is its depilatory action.[84] Long exposures of the head will most surely result in a circumscribed baldness, corresponding to the side of the head exposed to the tube.

A peculiarity is that the hair so affected does not fall

---

80 See report of sixty-nine cases of X ray injuries. Dr. N. Stone Scott, American X Ray Journal, August, 1897.

81 British Medical Journal, Nov. 7, 1896.

82 Philadelphia Polyclinic, Dec. 12, 1896.

83 New York Medical Times. Dr. Gage on "Erythema Following Exposure to X Rays."

84 "See X Rays a Depilatory." Dr. Freund, Magazine of Medicine, August, 1897.

out at once; but in two weeks or more the area so affected will suddenly and without any premonitory symptoms become quite bald. Even the fine lanugo hairs may vanish. This effect seems to be an electrical one, but I believe it strengthens the emissions or molecular bombardment theory of Tesla. It is possible that by the bombardment of the material atoms heat is produced, which burns or loosens the hair in its follicle. I have heard of only two such cases, but only one seems to have been recorded.[85] The subject in this case was exposed for forty minutes to the rays and temporary baldness, or *alopecia areata radiosa,* lasting several months resulted. I have no doubt as to the cause of the condition in this case, and only attribute it to the action of the rays. I believe that by the employment of some di-electric, such as an oil or unguentum, which is rich in fat, will prevent this depilatory action; however, suffice it to say that an exposure of twenty minutes, directly of the head (uncovered), should be the limit. I may say here that the alopecia so resulting was not permanent. The hair returned readily and grew rapidly under stimulating treatment.

The lenses of the eye, aided by the constant moisture of the salty secretion of the lachrymal gland, are to a great extent impervious to the rays, but exposure of the eyes is often accompanied by pain, felt in and about the eyes, after working for a length of time with the rays.

The rays seem to have a warming effect upon the brain, causing first anxiety and later drowsiness, followed by sleep. The person exposed seems to lose all thought of time or monotony, and is usually surprised to find that a certain length of time has elapsed; whether this is due to a direct action of the rays upon the brain itself, or to the constant

---

85 Kolle: Brooklyn Medical Journal, December, 1896; Electrical Engineer, March 10, 1897; American X Ray Journal, August, 1897.

buzzing or humming of the rheotome, I am as yet unable to say.

IN GEOLOGY AND MINERALOGY.

In geology and mineralogy the rays have been applied to some extent, and one of the earliest discoveries was that diamonds were comparatively pervious to these rays,[86] and that in this way genuine stones could be quickly distinguished from the artificial ones, as the latter were highly opaque to the rays and gave denser shadows than the real gem.

This in itself is of considerable importance to those handling gems, as they can quickly determine between the two, by the use of the fluoroscope or optic method. The stones furthermore need not necessarily be removed from their settings for this method of examination.

IN MINING.

In mining the rays have been utilized in defining free gold in quartz, and the results obtained by Dr. J. C. Perry, etc., speak highly of the value of the rays, the latter "showed the valuable metal as plainly as if it lay on the surface of the quartz."

IN BOTANY.[87]

In botany magnificent results have been attained. By the optic method (use of the screen), or the graphic method (using the photographic plate), the minute details of plant life can be observed and recorded. The details of the various forms of the organs of vegetation, its embryo,

86 Buquet & Gescord: "Action of the X Rays upon the Diamond and its Imitations," Comptes Rendus, Feb. 24, 1896; Thompson, S. P.: The Electrician, London, May 18, 1896.

87 See Hinterberger: "Roentgenogramme von Pflanzentheilen," Wied. Annalen, 1897.

phytomer, caulicle, cotyledons, seed-leaves, ascending and descending axis, etc., the plumule of the seed may be differentiated. as well as the monocotyledonous from the poly or diaotyledonous embryos; the roots and their many peculiarities can be studied and recorded by the graphic method, in fact the tedious and expensive drawings, perfect only to a degree, are at once replaced by the perfect and accurate, and most interesting radiograms.

IN ZOOLOGY.

In zoology radiograms of living specimens replace those of the vivisected animal. In radiograms made from life, with proper exposure, the tissue outline and the relative position of the organs to the bony skeleton are represented in a true and exact manner. The specimen need not be dissected as heretofore, and the living animal can be examined without injury or inconvenience by the aid of the fluoroscope; the parts can be seen in life and the relation of the living organs to the bony frame may in this way be studied.

CONCLUSION.

In conclusion of the volume the contents of which I have but humbly presented to you, I might suggest a few of the possibilities in the use of the rays in the future.

In consideration of the fact that the rays are comparable to a great extent with the ultra-ultra-violet-light rays, there may be a possibility of treating disease, irrespective of nature, with happy result.

Indeed, we need hardly be surprised to hear of the general treatment, in the near future, of such diseases as tuberculosis, cancer, diphtheria, rheumatism, etc., and of its applicability to pharmacy (analytical).

M. Despeignes[88] gives a full report of a case of cancer treated with the X rays. He claims that the continued use of this treatment diminished the size of the tumor, and that at the time of the patient's death it was much smaller. He believes that the treatment ameliorated the general condition of the patient, prolonged life for fully two weeks, suppressed the pain absolutely, where opium and morphine had been given before in considerable quantity, in the region of the tumor, besides diminishing the size of the tumor and its growth.

Unfortunately the treatment in this case was commenced rather late in the disease; perhaps better or more promising results might have been obtained, had the patient been treated earlier.

---

88 Lyon Medical, Aug. 9, 1896.

In pharmacy Spanish saffron has been differentiated from the artificial variety by the aid of the rays.

The rays may be employed in the examination of foods, etc.,[89] or in the examination of the brain for tumors, foreign bodies or blood clots; for examination of the lungs, stomach, aided by the ingestion of some opaque liquid, kidneys, etc.

The rays can be used for the examination of metals such as armor plate, shells, cartridges, etc., or in determining the nature of suspicious packets supposed to contain an explosive or bomb.

Gunpowder is opaque to the rays, and the granular character of the same can be determined by the ragged edge observed along the walls of the receptacle which contains it, as in a radiogram made of an ordinary loaded gun cartridge.

But the most valuable of all will be its general use and further application in medicine and surgery, wherein humanity has been most benefited.

Thankfully may we accept the faithful efforts of Professor Roentgen and his many scientific followers, who have materially aided in advancing and perfecting his discovery —"*pro bono publico.*"

---

89 Ranwez, F.: "Application of X Rays to Analyze Vegetable Matter," Comptes Rendus, April 13, 1896.

BIBLIOGRAPHY.

American Electrician.
Electrical Engineer.
Electricity.
Science.
Scientific American.
Electrical Review, London.
Western Electrician.
Wiedemann's Annalen.
Wildermann's Electricitt.
Electrical World.
Electrical Review, New York.
Electricity and Its Modern Application (Trevet).
Tesla's Inv., Res. and Writings (Martin).
London Electrician.
Philosophical Magazine, London.
Comptes Rendus.
Electrische Zeitung.
L'Industrie Electrique.
Nuovo Cimento, Italy.
Encyclopedia Britannica.
International Encyclopedia.
Electricity in Electro-Therapy (Houston & Kennelly).
Sinusoidal Currents (F. W. Langdon, M. D.).
New York Medical Journal.
Philadelphia Polyclinic.
Medical Record, New York.
Wiener Medicinische Blatter.
Lyon Medical.
New York Medical Times.
British Medical Journal.
American Journal of Medicine.
American Journal of Medical Science.
Brooklyn Medical Journal.
Transactions of Brooklyn Surgical Society.
Cincinnati Lancet Clinic.
Proceedings of the Academia Medico Chirurgia di Perugia, Vol. III.
Practical Radiography (Ward, London).
Clinical Skiagraphy (Rowland, London).
Photography of the Invisible (Morton, New York).
X-Rays (Trevet).
Phenomena of the Anode and Cathode (Thomson).
Induction Coils (Norris).
Photogram (London).
American X Ray Journal.
Lectures on the X rays (Kolle).
Physics (Ganot).
Physics (Peck).
Chemistry (Fowne; Bartley).

THE END.

THE

Morton-Wimshurst-Holtz

INFLUENCE MACHINE.

FOR THERAPEUTICAL PURPOSES AND X-RAY WORK.

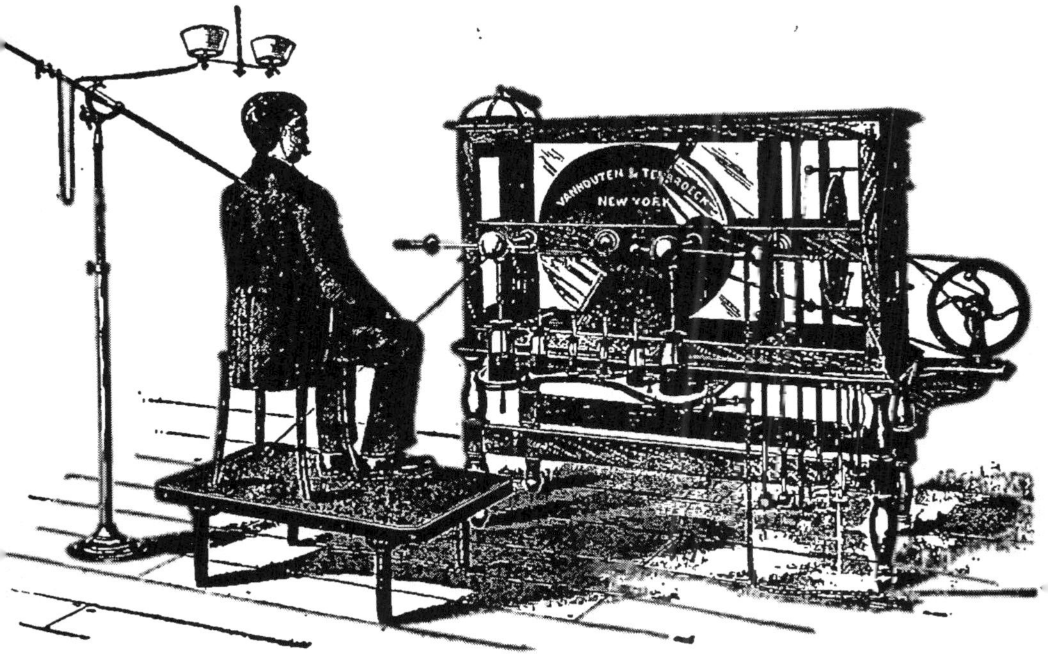

THE BEST IN THE WORLD.

Purchasers of our machine tell us that it is far superior to a coil for x-ray work, and its therapeutic properties are of inestimable value.

VAN HOUTEN & TEN BROECK,

300 FOURTH AVENUE, NEW YORK.

Makers of High-Grade Electro-Therapeutical Apparatus.

Write for X-Ray Catalogue and static literature.

X-RAY APPARATUS.

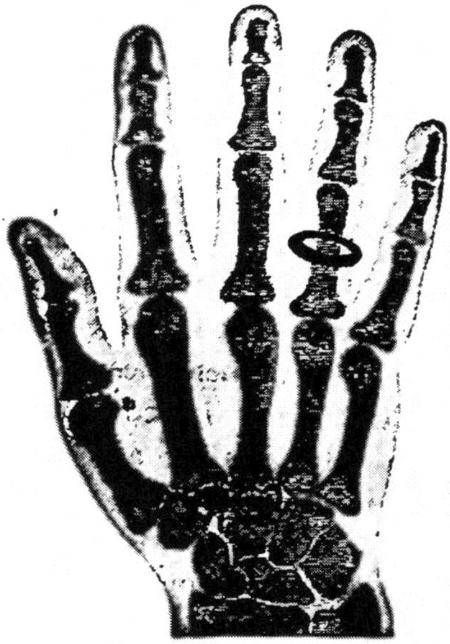

Self-Adjusting Focus Tubes,

Tube Stands,

Ruhmkorff Coils,

Adjustable Multiple Condensers,

Fluoroscopes and Screens,

Electric Motors with Make-and-Break Attachments,

X-Ray Dry Plates.

SEND FOR CATALOGUE.

Complete X-Ray Outfits for Radiography and Fluoroscopic Demonstration furnished for use with Primary Batteries, Storage Batteries, or the Electric Current.

E. B. Meyrowitz

Optician,

MANUFACTURER OF MEDICO-OPTICAL AND ELECTRO-SURGICAL APPARATUS.

104 E. Twenty-third Street, 125 W. Forty-second Street.

NEW YORK CITY.

ARC ELECTRIC LIGHT MAGIC LANTERN.

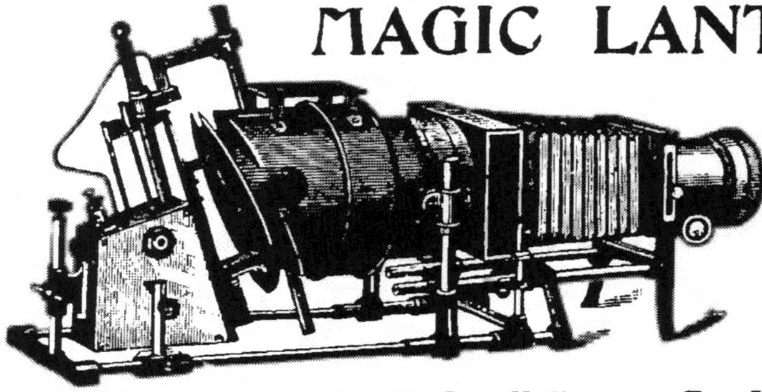

Parts removable for introduction of scientific attachments and various forms of light.

By special arrangement with Dr. Kolle we offer Lantern Slides from any of his X-Ray Negatives.

J. B. COLT & CO., (Dept. 6),
115-117 Nassau Street, New York,

Manufacturers of APPARATUS for the Production and Manipulation of LIGHT.

Also of LANTERN SLIDES and Other Accessories.

Send for CATALOGUE, and INFORMATION.

C. F. SPLITDORF,

MANUFACTURER OF

X-RAY COILS.

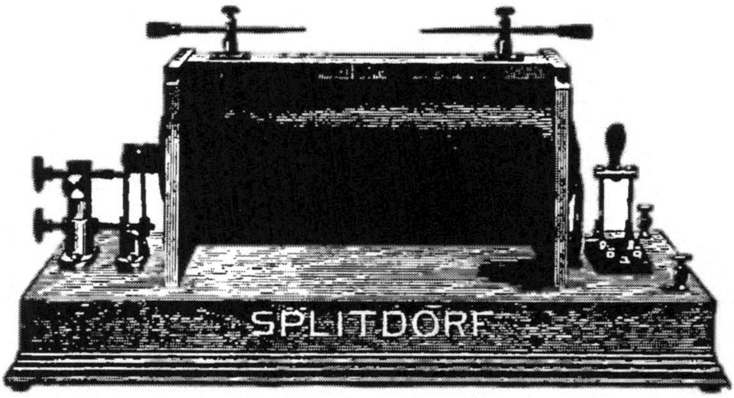

Medical Batteries, Electrodes, Ozone Generators, Galvanometers, and all Special Electrical Appliances for Physicians and Surgeons.

17-27 VANDEWATER STREET, - NEW YORK CITY.